Madness, Cannabis and Colonialism

Madness, Cannabis and Colonialism

The 'Native-Only' Lunatic Asylums of British India, 1857–1900

James H. Mills
Department of History
University College Northampton

First published in Great Britain 2000 by
MACMILLAN PRESS LTD
Houndmills, Basingstoke, Hampshire RG21 6XS and London
Companies and representatives throughout the world

A catalogue record for this book is available from the British Library.

ISBN 0–333–79334–X

First published in the United States of America 2000 by
ST. MARTIN'S PRESS, INC.,
Scholarly and Reference Division,
175 Fifth Avenue, New York, N.Y. 10010

ISBN 0–312–23359–0

Library of Congress Cataloging-in-Publication Data
Mills, James H., 1970–
Madness, cannabis and colonialism : the "native-only" lunatic asylums of British India, 1857–1900 / James H. Mills.
p.   cm.
Includes bibliographical references and index.
ISBN 0–312–23359–0
1. Mental illness—India—Treatment—History—19th century. 2. Asylums——India—History—19th century. 3. Insane—Commitment and detention—India——History—19th century. 4. Psychiatric hospitals—India—History—19th century.
I. Title.

RC451.I4 M556   2000
362.2'1'095409034—dc21

00–024948

This book is printed on paper suitable for recycling and made from fully managed and sustained forest sources.

10   9   8   7   6   5   4   3   2   1
09   08   07   06   05   04   03   02   01   00

Printed and bound in Great Britain by
Antony Rowe Ltd, Chippenham, Wiltshire

Contents

List of Figures and Tables

Figures

Tables

Acknowledgements

I owe thanks to a range of people and institutions for their help in completing this book. Special thanks are due to Dr Crispin Bates of the Department of History, Edinburgh University. He was a patient and energetic supervisor while I was completing the research that is the basis for this work and has since been a thoughtful and perceptive reader of the various drafts of this book.

Drs Paul Bailey and Ian Duffield at Edinburgh also deserve thanks for their help and support, as does Professor Roger Jeffery of the Department of Sociology there, who was the source of useful insights from a different perspective. Similarly, I am grateful to Dr Clare Anderson of Leicester University and Dr Cathy Coleborne of the University of Waikato, New Zealand, who have both offered encouragement while throwing in disruptive but irresistible ideas. Dr David Washbrook of St Antony's College, Oxford, Dr Steve Sturdy at the Science Studies Unit at Edinburgh and Professor David Arnold at SOAS have also been good enough to advise on various parts of this book.

The most important period of research for the whole project was that which I spent in India. I gratefully acknowledge the support of the British Academy, the Carnegie Trust for the Universities of Scotland and the George Scott Travelling Scholarship which made the trip possible, and the efforts of Dr Neeladri Bhattacharya of the Centre for Historical Studies at the Jawaharlal Nehru University in New Delhi, who secured my affiliation there. Many people helped me in India and the staff at the National Archives of India and at the State Archives of Uttar Pradesh deserve praise, as do those at the hospitals that I visited at Delhi, Agra and Bareilly. Special thanks are due to Professor Shridhar Sharma of the Hospital for Mental Diseases at Delhi for his information on mental health services in contemporary India and also to Dr Aditya Kumar of the Mental Hospital at Agra, who had personally preserved the unique set of case notes which is such an important and original source for this work and who made possible my stay in one of the very institutions that I was studying. I should also like to say thanks to the Ahuja family who were my hosts in New Delhi in 1995 and who

vii

did so much to make me feel like a welcome addition to their household.

In the UK the staff at the National Library of Scotland, the Edinburgh University Library and the Lothian Health Board Collection were always helpful, as were those at the India Office Library, the Wellcome Institute and the London School for Hygiene and Tropical Medicine. I should also like to thank the Department of History at University College Northampton which organised a sabbatical for me so as to give me time to complete the manuscript.

Above all though I want to thank Mum, Dad, Barney and Cary, my brother. Their total support and encouragement at all times have made the book possible. This is for the Mills family, with love.

JAMES H. MILLS

The illustrations on pages 55 and 123 are reproduced with the permission of the British Library.

List of Abbreviations

Ben.	Bengal
Bom.	Bombay
Civ.Asst.Surg.	Civil Assistant Surgeon
Civ.Surg.	Civil Surgeon
Comm.	Commissioner
C.Provs.	Central Provinces
GOI	Government of India
IGH	Inspector-General of Hospitals
IGP	Inspector-General of Prisons
IG Police	Inspector-General of Police
IHDC	Indian Hemp Drugs Commission
IMD	Indian Medical Department
LA	Lunatic Asylum
Mad.	Madras
Mag.	Magistrate
NWP	North-Western Provinces
Pres.	President
Sec.	Secretary
Super.	Superintendent

Note on Sources

Volume number	Patient number in volume	Date of admission
Case Book IA,	patient no.1,	admitted 1 January 1861.

The above is an example of the references in the footnotes made to the case notes of the Lucknow Lunatic Asylum (see Acknowledgements and Bibliography for details). The reference is to which of the volumes contains the case note (the original numbering on the three surviving volumes is IA, II and IV and this has been retained), to the patient number within that volume and the date on which that patient was admitted according to the information available on the case note.

Introduction

> The very obnoxious practice of masterbation [sic] which is the cause of insanity in many cases, and which aggravates the disease, is very common amongst the inmates of the asylum here. I have perplexed myself about the vice and in former years endeavoured to prevent it by blistering the penis with crotenal etc., but without effect, and various medicines were given in vain with the view of moderating or repressing the desire.
>
> During the past year I have tried Dr Yellowless's mode of prevention very recently practiced in asylums at home, and so far as it has gone, I am very much satisfied with the result.
>
> The suggestion was founded on the anatomical fact that the prepuce was anatomically necessary for the erection of the penis. Its anatomical use was to give a cover for the increased size of the organ. If you prevented the prepuce going to that use, you would make erections so painful that it would be practically impossible, and emissions therefore unlikely.
>
> The operation is very simple: the prepuce at the very root of the glans is pierced with an ordinary silver needle, the ends of which are tied together.[1]

The report of the superintendent in charge at the asylum in Rangoon to the Government of India on the administration of that institution during 1877 included the above confession. The superintendent had been using extreme violence in his treatment of those in his charge in order to impose his own notions of correct sexual behaviour. This did not simply involve him seeking to stop the inmates' masturbation. He was trying to stop them from wanting to masturbate; in his words his techniques were devised 'with the view of moderating or repressing the desire'.

Yet of course the above account is not a confession and it brought no censure from his superiors. In fact his inclusion of the account in a routine report on his duties at the asylum shows that he considered his actions to be very much part of those duties and that by including the above details in a summary of his proceedings

1

he would be proving to those reading the report that he was taking his role at the asylum seriously and tackling it diligently. In other words the violence visited upon the Indians at the asylum was state sanctioned. In the asylums of British India in the 1870s the colonial government seems to have established sites where its officers could intervene in the lives of those that the state had chosen to incarcerate in an attempt to reorder their psyches by altering not just what they did but what they wanted to do.

The above account also suggests however that the power of the Government of India and its institutions was often resisted. The superintendent after all admits that he resorted to needles and ties after the failure of other techniques that he experimented with to have an impact on the behaviour of those that he was seeking to change. But it is not at all clear how to interpret Indian masturbation as resistance in a British-run lunatic asylum, especially in an asylum where the chief medical officer was seeking to prohibit such behaviour. It could be possible to see this continued defiance of the doctor's painful attempts to impose his moral order as heroic, the resort to 'weapons of the weak'[2] on the part of the subjected. These inmates may have lost their freedom as they were incarcerated in a colonial institution but they were determined to resist the imposition of an alien order on their bodies.

Their status as 'insane' however raises other possibilities. Throughout this study there is a constant questioning of the nature of this label both in the development of nineteenth century psychiatry and medicine and in the shifting contexts of British India. At no point will this study accept the diagnosis of any of the inmates of the asylums of British India as 'insane'. This would simply be complying with the power relations of the period and colluding with the colonial approach of condemning or ignoring the statements and actions of those incarcerated in the asylums as unworthy of serious consideration. As shall be demonstrated these statements and actions are full of significance.

Constant masturbation is rarely acceptable in any society however and the motivations of the men in the account above, while not to be dismissed as simply 'mad', may have been so personal to the individuals involved that they were not communicable or comprehensible even to themselves. It may well have been highly individual and complex combinations of drives, demons and desires that compelled these men to masturbate rather than a determination to defy the medical officer's brutal agenda. As such their actions can be seen as resistance in the broadest sense, in as much as they served to frustrate the doctor's programme of controlling his inmates' sexuality. But the dogged masturbation might not have been a 'weapon of the weak' and it may well be that unfathomable pressures drove the men rather than a conscious determination to resist the doctor's designs. What inspired these men to carry on masturbating through the pain and to persist in 'perplexing' the medical officer may well have been drives utterly unconnected with the medical officer and his institution.

Ultimately however it is impossible to know what drove these men to masturbation because of the silences and the discourses of the records. If two of the issues to be developed in this study then are those already mentioned, the intentions of the British in establishing the lunatic asylums in India and the ways in which locals interacted with these institutions, then the third issue to be considered is the nature of the records left behind by these institutions. The account above is constructed in such a way as to represent masturbation as a 'vice' and the mutilation of genitals as rational. This does not necessarily reflect a natural moral order and would seem to reveal more about the obsessions of the British medical officer than it does about the 'insanity' of the inmates. The knowledge generated at the asylums had its own power then, the power to construct standards of normality and deviancy and of morality and immorality. This knowledge, contained in the array of case notes and official reports from British India available in the archives of England, Scotland and India will therefore also be considered in this study. The ideas constructed in these documents go some way to explaining not just how British officers thought about sanity and insanity in India, but how they thought about themselves in India and indeed how they thought about India itself.

Colonial history and the history of psychiatry

By looking at the asylums of British India from 1857 to about 1900 this study engages with both the historiographies of colonial history and of the history of psychiatry. In considering these three issues, of the knowledge generated at the asylums, of the Government of India's intentions in establishing the asylum system and of the reasons for and effects of Indian interactions with that system, this study intends to extend debates which have developed within both fields.

For example, the interest in the nature of the knowledge available at the asylums stems from the concerns with the issue of the productive property of language which can be found within both the historiographies of colonial and of medical history. These concerns have a common root in the general misgivings about the nature of language which doubt the modern conviction that language is simply 'a perpetual and objectively based correlation of the visible and the expressible.'[3] Critics of this naive understanding point out instead that language has a creative and productive power, 'language in texts always . . . functions ideationally in the representation of experience and the world.'[4]

Subaltern Studies writers like Ranajit Guha and Shahid Amin began in the 1980s to explore the productive nature of language in the records of colonial government. Ranajit Guha cited the broad range of primary sources that contain information on peasant rebellions from 'the exordial letter, telegram, despatch and communiqué to the terminal summary, report, judgement and proclamation'[5] as well as those secondary sources such as the reminiscences or retrospective accounts of administrators. While these accounts often conflict in their avowed purpose or in the information they contain on specific events, Guha pointed out that they were all written in what he variously calls the 'prose' or 'code of counter-insurgency'. In this code, an Islamic puritan becomes a *fanatic*, and revolt against the landlord becomes *defying the authority of the state*. While the record of events may often appear confused in these documents the intention in their being written in this way is not. The various sources are all acting to produce representations of actors and actions which justify the intervention of the colonizers. The accounts do this by portraying those defying the colonial state as politically illegitimate. As Guha concludes, 'these documents make no sense except in terms of a code of pacification which, under the Raj, was a complex of coercive intervention by the State and its protégés, the native elite, with arms and words.'[6]

Shahid Amin examined legal documents in colonial India and pointed out the paradox that 'historians of colonial India have hitherto, by and large, coupled their political opposition to pronouncements made by English judges on the "native" accused with an uncritical reading of judgements.'[7] The judgement passed on civil disturbances at Chauri Chaura appears to satisfactorily explain the criminal acts of the crowd. It concluded that their picketing of liquor and meat shops is to be blamed on the prices charged by the shopkeepers. However, this record slyly turns a Hindu/Muslim declaration of unity (based on the issues of temperance and vegetarianism) charged through with religious and political implications, into a simple act of wanton criminality by a typical mob. The economistic explanation entered in the records is formed within a colonial political discourse, where the demonstration of dissent is emptied of political significance by the act of recording the causes as economic. As Amin concludes: 'An economistic reading of the evidence did not yield a politics of the accused, but it has of the judgement itself.'[8] Colonial writing in these accounts is not transparently recording events. Rather it is producing new objects, images and ideas, which reflect and reproduce colonial ways of seeing and thinking about India.

Historians who consider medical documents rather than those who examine colonial records similarly explore this productive power of language and claim that medical documents, rather than offering objective scientific data, instead create 'a set of social messages wrapped up in technical language.'[9] Those who have studied psychiatric records in particular show how such case notes serve to produce their own stories which verify male fantasies of domination[10] or doctors' fantasies of efficacy.[11]

Chapters 1 and 2 will take up this issue of the productive nature of knowledge which has been discussed by historians of both colonialism and medicine. Chapter 1 will look at the assessments recorded of the patients' states of mind and the impressions given of the impact of the doctors' interventions in the case notes available for the asylums of British India. The chapter will consider whether these are accurate and objective clinical observations or constructed representations which are the result of the imaginings and attitudes of the British staff at the asylums. If the latter is the case then the nature of these imaginings and attitudes and what they tell the historian about the mindsets of the colonizers will be considered.

While Chapter 1 looks at what the case notes tell the historian about the way that knowledge was generated at the asylums, Chapter 2 considers the significance of that knowledge once those outside of the asylum began to take an interest in it. This chapter traces the way in which the information gathered in the asylums in the 1870s itself acted to generate further ideas, in this case the concept of the cannabis smoker as a threat to social order in India. This idea ended up being discussed in the House of Commons in the 1890s and indeed led to the establishment of the parliamentary

Indian Hemp Drugs Commission of 1893/4. This chapter concludes that in reality cannabis smoking was a widespread leisure and medicinal practice in nineteenth century India and those that used it constituted no great menace to British law and order. However the lack of knowledge about the subject population led the British administration in India to attach significance to any information that it was supplied with, even if this was information from as questionable a source as a lunatic asylum. As such the administrative expedient of blaming insanity on cannabis in the asylums of the 1870s was able eventually to lead to a parliamentary commission into the issue of cannabis use and the intervention of the British colonial state to prohibit cannabis use in parts of Indian society.

The British created knowledges about Indians in the asylums which reflected the position of judgement that they had assumed over inmates as doctors caring for the ill and as colonizers surveilling the colonized. Quite simply, power produced knowledge. Yet power manifested itself in other ways at the asylum, and both historians of medicine and those who have examined encounters in colonial contexts have considered the ways in which medical institutions and policies impacted on lives and on societies. Chapters 3 and 4 will consider these debates and look at the disciplinary functions of the asylums. This concern reflects an awareness of both the disciplinary functions of the psycho-sciences during the nineteenth century in the Western experience and the attempts at reordering and regulating populations which have been identified as central to the concerns of governments established by the West in its modern colonies.

The disciplinary functions of the psycho-sciences were first highlighted by Michel Foucault in his classic work on insanity in Western culture, *Madness and Civilization*.[12] This account has it that the origins of the asylum were as an institution where errant individuals identified as such by bourgeois morality[13] could be confined as punishment and be reformed. The walls of confinement enclosed 'fortresses of moral order . . . in which were taught religion and whatever was necessary to the peace of the state.'[14]

According to Foucault, by 1800 the doctor had taken on the responsibility for the reformatory procedures within the 'walls of confinement', so that 'what we call psychiatric practice is a certain moral tactic contemporary with the end of the eighteenth century, preserved in the rites of asylum life and overlaid by the myths of positivism.'[15] The asylum is a disciplinary site and the psychiatric practices were disciplinary techniques, where surveillance, judgement, patriarchy and physical coercion were combined and focused on the individual to 'impose in a universal form, a morality that will prevail from within upon those who are strangers to it.'[16]

Subsequent studies of the psycho-disciplines have confirmed their disciplinary functions. Andrew Scull identifies two stages in the development of the psycho-sciences in Britain and America which reflect alternative approaches to the disciplinary task:

> There is an abandonment of external coercion (which could never do more than force the crudest and least stable forms of outward conformity) for an approach that promises to produce the internalization of the necessary moral standards, by inducing the mad to collaborate in their own recapture by the forces of reason.[17]

In the same vein feminist writers emphasize the function of the psycho-sciences in disciplining the female sex, Elaine Showalter identifying 'the Darwinian nerve-specialist', who 'arose to dictate proper feminine behaviour outside the asylum as well as in it, to differentiate treatments for 'nervous' women of various class backgrounds, and to oppose women's efforts to change the conditions of their lives.'[18] Yannick Ripa who writes on the French experience concludes that 'this new "alienist" medicine flirted with religion, morality and the police; in a sense it became the keeper of the public order.'[19] She stresses that

> the asylum sought to force women back into the mould from which they had just tried to escape. Sick from lack of attention and understanding, women were supposed to be 'cured' without being either heard or understood. Behind the paternalistic philanthropy of the asylum there lurked violent forms of therapy whose aim was to silence women ... Alienist science as applied to women was at its birth a socially coercive form of medicine.[20]

Indeed, studying psychology in England from 1869 to 1939, Nikolas Rose concludes that what the various strands of theory and practice 'made possible was a scientific technique for the administration of individuals and populations in terms of their mental attributes and capacities.'[21] Quite simply, the psycho-sciences provided the means not only for disciplining individuals but also for disciplining, that is managing and governing, whole societies.

Historians who have looked at methods of government in contexts where Westerners were attempting to impose their authority over non-Western societies have similarly emphasized that medical techniques could be important in the process of assertion. Franz Fanon, himself a Western-trained psychiatrist, identified medicine as central to projects of imposing control in Africa. He asserted that the doctor was implicated in the disciplinary machinery of the colonial state and that 'the colonized perceives the doctor, the engineer, the school teacher, the rural constable through the haze of an almost organic confusion.'[22] Others have concluded that Fanon was right to see medicine in this way, Roy MacLeod stating that 'the history of medicine in empire refers to the . . . history of medical regimes as participants in the expansion and consolidation of political rule.'[23]

Various case studies provide the evidence for such conclusions. In India and Africa population movement was controlled in the name of medicine,[24] while there are instances where surveillance and detention of the colonized was authorized with reference to medical measures.[25] India also provides interesting examples where behaviour was regulated after the introduction of sanitation projects.[26] Those populations over which Europeans attempted to assert control were watched, controlled and reordered by medicine.

Indeed, the place of the psycho-sciences in particular in the disciplinary projects of colonial medicine has recently been explored in certain case studies. In Australia, Cathy Coleborne concludes that in the nineteenth century, 'the preservation of social order remained paramount in the intentions of the legislators in early Australia where lunacy was concerned.'[27] Sally Swartz identifies the unemployed members of the colonized population as of special concern to the authorities in the Cape Colony and finds the 'loose native', the non-working vagrant member of the urban masses, a regular admission to the Valkenberg asylum.[28]

Surprisingly little attention has been paid to the Asian experience. Lee's article on the asylums of Singapore is simply a descriptive account of their development ending with the conclusion that 'the conditions at Singapore, which was considered a "remote outpost" were not too bad, and her doctors and leading citizens enlightened men.'[29] Waltraud Ernst's *Mad Tales from the Raj* deals only with asylums for the European insane in British India before 1858. It does however offer the interesting point that even when focusing on the Western population in colonial contexts the psycho-sciences acted to discipline, in this case labelling as mad those likely to tarnish the reputation of the British in order to have them removed from the colony.[30]

The place of the psycho-sciences in the disciplinary projects of the British in colonial India will therefore be investigated here in two chapters. Chapter 3 locates the asylum alongside the police and prison systems detailed elsewhere[31] in the matrix of institutions and policies devised by the government in India to control the population and limit its mobility and perceived volatility. Chapter 4 examines how the regime inside the asylum was designed to give the medical officer command of the incarcerated Indian's body and behaviour so that that body and behaviour might be remoulded and produced to be efficient and obedient. In other words these two chapters focus on the place of the psycho-sciences in disciplining India on the macro-level, that is on the level of governing whole populations, and in disciplining India on the micro-level where individual Indian bodies were seized and drilled.

Chapters 5 and 6 however reflect the concern of historians who have worked either with the history of psychiatry or with the history of encounters in colonial contexts which was mentioned when considering the account of the superintendent of the Rangoon asylum earlier. This concern is with the way in which the intentions and projects of the authorities which establish institutions like the asylums are resisted, frustrated and ignored by those in and around those institutions.

This issue is often simplified into a study of 'resistance'. For example, in studies of patients opposing the definitions and practices of the psycho-disciplines this tends to be the emphasis. Roy Porter points to autobiography as one method of resisting the discourses of psychiatry as it allows a space for self-definition.[32] Autobiography is also a theme developed by Jann Matlock in her discussion of the French asylum patient Hersilie Rouy.[33] For Yannick Ripa, resistance to internment took four different forms:

> First, there was clearly expressed opposition which came in the form of a letter complaining about the committal; next came rebellion against the authorities; then escapes and attempted escapes; finally, general misbehaviour which expressed their feelings but affected the inmates themselves – for example, mutism and attempted suicide.[34]

Cheryl Krasnick Warsh similarly identifies letter writing, escape and suicide as instances of resistance in the Canadian Homewood Retreat but also points to violent and disruptive behaviour, all too easily disguised by the authorities as symptoms of an illness rather than as coherent expressions of anger, as behaviour indicating opposition to the situation in the asylum.[35] Indeed madness itself has been interpreted as resistance, where behaviour which refuses to conform to that expected is given the label 'insane' so as to justify disciplinary action and to discourage others from adopting that approach. This is an argument advanced in a number of feminist accounts of madness, Phyllis Chesler for example claims that women in American mental institutions in the nineteenth century did no more than behave in ways which defied male imposed norms of female propriety.[36]

Colonial studies though emphasize the perils of only looking for resistance when considering the responses of the subjected, as this accepts that the subjected can only express themselves in opposition to something, on grounds and in situations defined by others. For example the Subaltern Studies project identifies the politics of the lower classes as an 'autonomous domain' in the power relations of colonial India which 'far from being destroyed or rendered virtually ineffective, as was elite politics of the traditional type by the intrusion of colonialism . . . continued to operate vigorously in spite of the latter.'[37] Nicholas Thomas also develops this theme, exploring the possibility that '"natives" often had relatively autonomous representations and agendas, that might have been deaf to the enunciations of colonialism, or not so captive to them that mimicry seemed a necessary capitulation.'[38]

The actions and agendas of the patients in the Indian asylums will be considered then in Chapter 6. It needs to be emphasized that it is the interaction of the non-elite members of Indian society with medical institutions which will be the focus. Superintendents frequently made comments similar to the following about asylum admissions: 'The three classes whence the largest number are received are ryots, servants and beggars.'[39] The evidence on the case notes from the Lucknow lunatic asylum confirms this, as the usual entries under occupation are 'beggar', 'labour' [sic], and 'cultivator' and where caste information is given low-status categories like 'chumar'[40] and 'ahir'[41] are common. In other words it seems that the asylum was dealing with subaltern groups in Indian society and it is the interaction of such groups with the colonial institutions which will be considered.

The patient population is not the only group whose actions will be explored at the asylum as Indians interacted with the institutions in a number of roles. The majority of the staff was Indian, working in various capacities from that of sub-assistant surgeon to orderly to sweeper and gardener. In other words, it was not just the patients in the asylum who were encountering these institutions and who were capable of acting in ways that frustrated or negotiated the intentions of those who established the asylums.

The evidence also suggests that members of the local community were not simply passive participants in the asylum system in India, as patients or internees gathered in by disciplinary practice. Many seem to have actively sought to interact with the asylum by seeking admission for themselves and for members of their friends or family while pursuing the release of others. Their agendas in dealing with the asylum are important, as they point to the possibility that it was not simply the authorities that had the power to define what these institutions should act as and be used for. It is the interaction of the community around the asylums with those institutions that will be the subject of Chapter 5.

The asylums of British India

From a very early date there is evidence that the British decided that a specialist facility needed to be available to them in which they could segregate those they encountered in the Indian population as insane. In 1795 the Commander in Chief of the Bengal Army wrote to the Governor General proposing to establish a 'house' at Monghier in which mad sepoys could be incarcerated.[42] At the time there were three such soldiers locked up in the guard room at the invalid depot in that garrison, a state of affairs the Commander considered highly unsuitable. The Governor-General's response was very positive as he agreed that this was all a good idea and sanctioned a facility to be designed for the reception of about twenty patients which could be expanded further should there be the demand.[43]

Just over 85 years later it was announced that, 'the asylum at Hazaribagh was closed in the month of March.'[44] Coming soon after the decision to put the Moydapore institution into mothballs,[45] the expansion of the asylum system for those the British considered mad and wished to incarcerate amongst the Indian population effectively ended and a period followed when new asylums were no longer planned and the numbers of those detained levelled off in the institutions which did remain. It is the twenty three years immediately preceding the publication in 1880 of the decision to close the Hazaribagh asylum which will broadly be the focus of this study.

The reason that the period 1857 to 1880 is important is not simply that it was the first years of direct rule of India by the British after the dissolution of the East India Company. The period was the most significant in the history of asylum provision for Indians by the British in the nineteenth century.

For example, in the realm of law it was a period of important activity. Act XXXVI of 1858 was the first act specifically designed to provide a legal framework for incarcerating those Indians considered mad by the British who had not come to the attention of the authorities through criminal behaviour. The legal provisions for criminal lunatics of the various administrations of India were also standardized in Chapter XXVII of the Criminal Procedure Code which was passed in 1861.

While the British in this period were establishing a legal framework in which those Indians they considered mad could be dealt with, they were also setting up an institutional network in which those Indians could be detained. With the opening of the Lucknow Lunatic Asylum in 1859 there began two decades of unprecedented activity in providing buildings to contain those the British encountered as 'mad' in the Indian population. Of the twenty-six asylums which operated in the areas under the jurisdiction of the Government of India in this period no less than sixteen have their origins in the 1860s and 1870s.[46] Alongside this building of new asylums the institutions which pre-dated the period 1857 to 1880 were the subject of expansion programmes, so that reports such as that for the Dacca Asylum in 1875 were common:

> The Construction of cells has been sanctioned by His Honor the Lieutenant Governor, and will be carried out at a cost not exceeding Rs. 21500. . . . This new building will consist of 20 cells capable of accommodating 40 lunatics, two in each cell, on the plan of the present female ward.[47]

This host of new buildings was quickly pressed into use and it was in this period that the number of detainees in institutions designated 'lunatic asylums' made the most significant leaps of the nineteenth century. Just looking at the asylum population figures of the three Presidencies demonstrates the importance of the period. In 1865 in the asylums of the Bombay Presidency there were 353[48] inmates at the end of the year, by 1875 there were 568[49] and by 1880 646.[50] The asylum population grew by some 83 per cent in the fifteen year period until 1880, leaping 60 per cent in the decade between 1865 and 1875 alone. In the fifteen years after 1880 though the asylum population grew by just 10 per cent.[51] In Madras the population of the asylum was just 140[52] people in 1867, but by 1880 this had more than doubled to 330.[53] This period of significant growth continued until 1885 when the asylum population reached 600[54] people at which point it seems to have virtually stopped growing, peaking in the nineteenth century at 608[55] in 1895 before falling to 559[56] in 1900.

It was in the Bengal Presidency, which had the most asylums of any one administration in India and in which the most people were incarcerated as 'lunatics' that the story of this period is most clearly told. In 1865 the total population of all the asylums was 627 people which by 1875 had risen to 1147,[57] a growth of 82 per cent in ten years. This was a peak in the nineteenth century as ten years later the population was 955[58] and by 1900 the population had fallen to 906.[59]

As is evident from such figures this was hardly the 'great incarceration' of people in which the asylum has been implicated in the nineteenth-century European context. Figures available for 1880 suggest that there were only around 2750 patients incarcerated for the whole of India at the end of a period of rapid expansion and after which rates of growth in the asylum population slowed to a trickle or even turned negative.[60] What will be explored here then is not a series of institutions which contained a significant proportion of the Indian population. It is the burst of energy in the provision of facilities for those that the British decided were 'lunatic' in the two decades or so after they took direct control of the government of India in 1857 that needs explaining and which promises to bring into focus the concerns and contemplated projects of the British in India in such an important period.

The study however does extend itself to the end of the century in considering the Indian Hemp Drugs Commission. As already mentioned this was the parliamentary commission established by the House of Commons in 1893/4 to investigate the issue of cannabis use in the population of India. It will be demonstrated that the network of asylums which was expanded and established in this burst of governmental energy in the 1860s and 1870s was capable of producing ideas and information which were to become powerful enough to transcend the domain of colonial government and to become an issue for the metropolitain government of Britain.

1

The Asylum Archive: the Production of Knowledge at the Colonial Asylum

Tracing the time and effort expended in the early 1870s on deciding the form of the end of year statistical report demonstrates the importance attached to the collection and compilation of information at the asylum. The Inspector-General of Hospitals in the Indian Medical Department in Calcutta effected a series of reforms in the report in Bengal early in the decade. Circular Memorandum No. 105 of 1871 included the note: 'The Inspector-General of Hospitals observes that some diversity exists in the forms of Statistical Returns of Lunatic Asylums. As it is essential, for purposes of comparison and compilation, that these forms shall be uniform, the following illustrations of those which should be invariably appended to the Annual Report have been prepared.'[1] There followed a list of sixteen tables which were to be produced by each asylum in the end of year report. The previous year the Cuttack asylum had submitted thirteen tables, the Moydapore institution had included only nine in its report and so on. The new system was to standardize the way that information was presented on issues which had previously been tabulated in different ways by the various asylums, issues such as the type of madness diagnosed. It also insisted on statistical representations being produced on issues that had not previously been considered in such a form, issues such as the rates of mortality compared to duration of residence.

It was subsequently suggested in 1872 that these forms should be adopted by the Government of India for all the asylums under its jurisdiction. In forwarding copies of his new tables the Inspector-General explained:

It is desirable in the first place that I should indicate clearly the objects and uses which these forms are intended to subserve. Their main object is to exhibit- *firstly*, the condition under which insanity arises among a community; and *secondly*, the circumstances and appliances under which recovery from insanity occurs. A knowledge of these conditions and circumstances is necessary for the adoption of means towards the prevention and cure of insanity and the more carefully and systematically they are noted and exhibited the more power we possess in both directions.[2]

His forms were not accepted by all and the ensuing controversy was settled by the referral of the matter to a committee in 1873. The Government of India received the committee's opinions and tinkered with its suggestions and finally a Resolution was passed in 1874.[3] However this Resolution only offered the chosen tables as the suggested standard and did not impose them as the expected norm and asylums certainly chose to continue with their own preferred systems.[4]

Because of the significance attached at the time to information at the asylum there is an extensive set of records available to the historian for exploring the asylums of British India. These records will be examined in two parts. The first, which concerns this chapter, will look at the nature of the data collected. Considering the accuracy of the information and the types of information found in these documents leads on to a assessment of what historians might use the documents produced by colonial medical institutions to investigate. The second part, which forms the next chapter, will look at the way in which the asylum acted as a site where knowledge of India was generated to be fed into the wider systems of colonial government through the medium of statistics.

Statistical analysis, retrospective diagnosis and discourse analysis

A variety of texts survives from the psychiatric institutions of British India. This includes the end of year reports with detailed statistical tables enumerating information on all matters from the number of patients in each religious group to the average cost per patient. Also available are individual patient case notes on which the details of what the doctor has observed of the individual patient are recorded and lengthy articles in professional journals in which theoretical matters are discussed and strange symptoms recorded. This all seems fairly standard material for asylums after 1850 the world over, and a number of accounts have used such sources in an attempt to reconstruct the asylum experience of the nineteenth-century.[5]

The first approach to these sources in many of these accounts is the exhaustive collation of the statistical data available for a specified series of years to establish information on the number of patients treated in each age group, the duration of stay, the numbers diagnosed under each type of madness and so on. In other words the first approach is an attempt to create a statistical profile of the patient population.[6] The second approach is retrospective diagnosis, where the appropriate late twentieth century label is applied to the symptoms recorded in the case notes of the past. This latter exercise is designed to reveal what types of mental illness, as understood by the more advanced and scientifically validated systems of today, were being treated in the hospitals of previous ages.[7]

The reasons why these approaches will not be accepted in this study will be considered first before explaining the methodology which will be adopted in this chapter.

Statistical analysis

Even if it were desirable to collate the information available and from it to build statistical pictures of the asylum population[8] there would be serious problems with any conclusions as it seems that the reliability of the data cannot be assumed. Simple data like the age of the patient was recorded on every case note and was collated in the tables of the end of year annual reports. The data collected in these tables was obviously scrutinized as it was often used as the basis for observations in the end of year reports:

> The tendency to insanity is most distinctly marked in the third and fourth decennia of life; it is less marked between the 40th and 60th years of age, still less marked under 20 years of age and reaches its minimum as old age advances.[9]

Yet serious doubts can be raised about the accuracy of the ages entered on the case notes. Of the 721 notes, 508 have ages which are entered as multiples of five. In other words about 70 per cent of the patients were entered as being 15, 20, 25, 30 and so on years old upon admission. This suggests that a process of estimation was at work on the part of the medical officer filling in the case note (or alternatively that there is a fearful correlation between insanity in nineteenth century Lucknow and reaching an age which is a multiple of five). Indeed, entries on some of the case notes seem to support the idea that an age was entered for a patient which might later be changed as more information became available or renewed attempts at estimation were made. Patient no. 110 in the first volume of case notes was admitted in May 1861 and discharged in January 1862.[10] He was judged to be 12 years old when the case note was first filled in and yet in the same box there is pencilled in the figure 18. He was not in the asylum for six years so this new figure does not reflect an attempt to record his age on discharge. Rather it shows a revision of the record of the man's age.

Lobha was admitted in August 1868 and died in November 1869. Originally judged to be 27 years old, a thick, black line through this figure suggests dissatisfaction with this information and a new figure of 50 was entered.[11] Not that age, when revised, was always revised upwards. Kovingbeebaree was admitted and discharged in the summer of 1864. It was originally recorded that he was 20 years old, an estimate that was eventually replaced with the figure 14.[12]

This process of estimation in deciding the age of patients admitted to the asylum does not seem limited to the Lucknow asylum or indeed to the 1860s and 1870s. It was pointed out in Bombay in 1874 for example that 'Deputy-Surgeon General Maitland objects to the tables . . . he also considers there will be difficulty in obtaining the age etc. of insanes.'[13] A small collection of case notes from the beginning of the twentieth century which was authored by a Dr Robertson-Milne in Bengal included that of Jabu Sheikh.[14] On his case note under the 'age' heading is the following entry:

40! (25!)

What age Jabu Sheikh was when inspected by the doctor is open to question, as is the age Dr Robertson-Milne thought him to be. What is clear though is that there was no definite information on this point and that a process of estimation was adopted, a process which in this case appears to have been frustrating the medical officer.[15] Data on more complex issues like cause of madness or even the type of madness that the patient was deemed to be suffering from is similarly problematic and cannot be taken as reliable information on reality. The problems of collecting information on the cause of madness will be discussed in an exploration of the issue of ganja smoking as assigned cause in Chapter 2. The difficulties in using the data on the type of madness diagnosed and treated in the asylums might be considered here though. In 1867 for example, Dr James

Table 1.1 Types of madness at the Dacca Lunatic Asylum in the year 1867

diagnosis	remained 31st Dec. 1866	admitted during the year 1867	total	males	females	total
amentia	1	0	1	1	0	1
dementia	73	9	82	65	17	82
mania acute	1	9	10	8	2	10
mania chronic	132	47	179	158	21	179
monomania	7	11	18	15	3	18
moral insanity	2	1	3	2	1	3
total	216	77	293	249	44	293

Source: Asylums in Bengal for the Year 1867, p. 60.

Wise, who was to go on and publish articles on insanity in India in professional journals,[16] included Table 1.1 in his end of year report on the Dacca asylum.[17]

From such a table it would be possible to conclude for example that most lunatics admitted to the Dacca asylum were chronic maniacs. The difficulty in using these statistics is that without knowing when 'mania', 'melancholia', 'dementia' and so on were applied as labels it would be impossible to understand what types of behaviour were being treated in the asylum.

Historians have invented various ways of overcoming this problem of understanding the types of behaviour signified by the labels in the statistical tables. Allan Beveridge reproduced the statistics at the Royal Edinburgh Asylum to discover that 'during Clouston's period of office the commonest clinical conditions identified using the traditional M.P.A. classification were those of mania and melancholia.'[18] Beveridge then included examples from the case notes that he claims are 'representative' of each mental state. For mania there is the example from the Edinburgh case notes of Andrew J. who is 'intensely excited'[19] and was 'talking incessantly'; for melancholia James S. is cited as he was suicidal[20] and so on. Anne Digby in her study of the York Retreat adopts a different way of making sense of the nineteenth century categories. After exhibiting a table of the diagnoses of first admissions between 1796 and 1843 she simply offers her own equivalents to the old labels: 'Manias and melancholy approximate broadly to manic-depressive illness: moral insanity to personality disorder; idiocy and imbecility to mental handicap; and dementia to dementia.'[21]

Such an approach is deeply problematic, certainly in the Indian instance, because of observations like the following from medical officers working in the asylums of the period:

> On the question of the nomenclature and the difficulties in the classifi-cation of some forms of mental diseases, the following careful note occurs in Dr Crombie's report – 'Every year references are made to the uncer-tainty of nomenclature in the hands of different Superintendents. As a matter of fact, there is room for difference of practice. The prevailing type of insanity in this part of India is that which is manifested by eccentricity, loquacity and general joyfulness and absurdity of demean-our, generally without delusions and with no loss of intelligence. These cases I class as chronic mania as they exhibit exaltation of the emo-tional faculties. But they often pass into a condition of chronic dementia when the emotional excitement becomes combined with diminished mental power. It is possible that one observer may classify such a case of chronic dementia, while another noticing the exaltation of emotion would en-ter it as one of chronic mania. The diagnosis between melancholia and dementia is not always easy. In both there is the same abstraction and disregard of surroundings, similar solitary habits and silence or reluc-tance to speak, and perhaps similar disregard of decency and personal cleanliness; but in one case these symptoms are due to the mind being so completely occupied by one thought of fear or misfortune or sorrow that it leaves no room for any other consideration, and in the other case the mental faculties are so degraded as to be incapable of being roused to an appreciation of what is taking place. On the other hand, the distinction between dementia and imbecility is dependent on the history of the case. If the mental degradation has occurred after the full development of the mental faculties it is a case of dementia; if it is due to arrest of development of the mental power in infancy it is a case of imbecility. The descriptive rolls on which the diagnosis depends are generally altogether worthless: they either contain no information whatever or are quite untrustworthy. Again, recurrent acute mania, whether that which follows epileptic attacks, or some unknown cause might, by one who regards chiefly the chronicity of the cause, which often lasts many years, be entered as chronic mania; while another having regard only to the acuteness of each individual attack would return it as acute ma-nia . . . In nature, the several types of insanity are not clearly defined: they dovetail, overlap and merge into one another, and as the case progresses the type of insanity often changes altogether.'[22]

In other words, in practice the label applied to a certain type of behaviour might vary considerably from asylum to asylum and from medical officer to medical officer. This doubt about diagnosis and classificatory systems is reflected in the variety of systems used in end of year reports. Dr Wise, writing in the same report as the one in which he included the above table, commented that:

> In his report on the Insane Asylums for 1866, Dr Green remarks upon the different classification of mental diseases followed in this asylum

from that adopted at Dullunda. On referring to the reports of former years, I find that Dr Simpson in 1862 distinguished between 9 varieties of insanity. In the reports for 1863 and 1864 8 classes only are enumerated; mania being subdivided into chronic and recurrent, and dementia into primary and secondary. In the report for 1865 only 5 classes are noted, mania chronic and dementia being made to include the subdivisions of former years. In 1866 the same nomenclature was followed. It has been found impossible to alter the classification of the present report as the monthly returns and case books have been filled in accordance with it.

It would be easy to adopt 'a uniform standard of distinction' in all asylums, but the orders on this subject are vague. The circular letter of the Medical Board no. 25, dated 13th July 1854 leaves it to the option of the Superintendents to follow one of two classifications; but it directs that if the minute subdivision is adopted, the varieties must be included under the 5 heads of moral insanity, monomania, mania and amentia. The table in the revised rules of 1860 only recognises these five divisions.[23]

What is clear in this passage is that problems with diagnosis and classification dated back at least to the 1850s and that attempts to impose a standard way of recording this data had failed. More remarkably it shows how the records of one asylum changed between doctors and year by year. Diagnosis and classification were issues in the 1850s and 1860s as much as in the 1880s and it should be noted from examples from other administrations in India that this was not a problem specific to the institutions in Bengal. In 1879 A.H.L. Fraser in the Central Provinces wrote in his overview of the asylum reports of the two institutions in that administration that:

As regards the types of insanity, there would appear to be considerable difference in the systems of classification observed. 'Chronic Mania' and 'Chronic Dementia' are credited with nearly two-thirds of the cases treated. In Nagpur 59 are set down to the former, and 35 to the latter, while in Jubbulpore the figures are 22 and 62 respectively. Similarly for 'acute mania' and 'acute dementia' the figures for Nagpur are 21 and 5, and those for Jubbulpore 7 and 11. Again 'idiotcy' of which no cases are recorded at Nagpur has 39 in the Jubbulpore asylum while 'melancholia' and 'insipientia' have far more cases in the former than in the latter institution.[24]

These problems with the meaning to be attached to each diagnostic category used render the statistics extremely problematic as counts of people suffering from specific conditions or behaving in specific ways. As is clear from Dr Crombie's lengthy account, the variety of classificatory systems which existed is the result of certain actions or appearances being included under different labels by different doctors. In other words there is no evidence that categories like 'mania' or 'melancholia' were stable ones. It is therefore impossible to be sure that one person to whom the label 'maniac' had been attached was behaving in the same way or exhibiting the same symptoms as another person from a different asylum, period or under the jurisdiction of another doctor to whom the label 'maniac' had similarly been attached. This is especially so when there was never a detailed attempt by the doctors involved to record their classificatory systems. In these circumstances it is not at all clear what a count of 179 'chronic maniacs' or 18 'monomaniacs' is actually a count of.

The annual reports of the asylums compiled statistical summaries of the year under the categories of information routinely gathered about the patients. The information under supposedly simple categories like that of the age of the patient is open to doubts about its accuracy and so any conclusions based on the statistical summaries of such data necessarily ignores all the evidence of inaccuracy and fabrication. More complex categories like that of type of mental illness suffered are similarly problematic as it is not at all clear what these categories refer to in clinical practice. In short, statistical profiling by historians of the patient population which involves the straightforward compilation of the available data into neat numerical summaries does no more than reproduce the loose and confused practices of the period when the information was originally collected.

Retrospective diagnosis

A number of studies of asylums from the past have concerned themselves with re-diagnosing the patients for whom case notes have survived. The new diagnoses rely on the information recorded on those documents. This process, of retrospective diagnosis, has most recently and consistently been employed by authors publishing in the *History of Psychiatry* journal. Rajendra Persaud studied the memorandum book of Samuel Coates between 1785 and 1825 and suggests that, 'schizophrenic symptoms were rare in 1790 and common in 1823.'[25] T. Turner also focused on the issue of schizophrenia as a historical phenomenon by attempting to assess the 'melancholy' and 'mopish' behaviours recorded on case records from as far back as the seventeenth century. He concluded the opposite of Persaud, that is that 'the historical evidence behind recency disease theories of schizophrenia seems thin.'[26] Using the information presented on the case notes as if it was an accurate record of symptoms these authors tried to establish whether schizophrenia is a condition of modernity or whether it is something that is a constant in human experience.

Other studies also mention schizophrenia in their conclusions although they are less interested in the 'recency' debate and more interested in assessing the types of illness as understood in today's psychiatric idiom for which patients were admitted to Victorian asylums. Parker, Sutta, Barnes and Fleet point out after work with the case notes from Rainhill that they 'decided to carry out a retrospective analysis of the diagnosis made in 1890 based on ICD9 and using all the clinical information available in the case notes'. They conclude that

> According to the retrospective diagnoses, depressive illness and schizophrenia comprised the largest categories, as they do today. Alcohol-related illnesses also account for a large number of diagnoses. Acute confusional states and personality disorders came next in order of diagnostic frequency, and acute confusional states were certainly diagnosed quite frequently. Patients with personality disorder, however, did not seem to be very often admitted to the Asylum. Schizo-affective psychosis and schizophreniform psychosis were not diagnoses included in the above list. This is probably a result of insufficient day-to-day clininal information being available from the notes.[27]

Allan Beveridge in his two part study of the Royal Edinburgh Asylum at the end of the nineteenth century analysed a sample of patient case notes according to the Research Diagnostic Criteria of Spitzer, Endicott and Robins (1975) and as such decided that 'it is apparent that organic illness featured prominently in the Asylum population, especially amongst West House patients... comparatively few patients met the criterion for schizophrenia although the numbers were higher for East House patients.'[28] As the quote from Parker *et al.* suggests, the authors using the retrospective diagnosis method are not unaware that there could be problems with the sources that they are using. 'Insufficient day-to-day clinical information' is suggested by these authors whereas elsewhere 'confusing past terminology'[29] is mentioned as a potential hazard for those wishing to diagnose from old case notes. The possibility that documents from asylums of the past may record 'madness' expressing itself in ways which would have been meaningful to physicians of that period and culture but which are less intelligible to people from outside that period and culture is a concern of T.H. Turner. As such he advises that, 'care must be taken in the use of modern operational criteria, based on first-rank symptoms and research-based assessments, for diagnosing psychotic illness from historical accounts.'[30]

However, despite these worries and the vague concerns expressed in such statements as 'we hope that our notes in 1990 were considerably more objective in their nature and considerably less Dickensian in their style'[31] the authors who use retrospective diagnosis as a historical method remain content to accept that the details on the case notes are clinical facts from which medical judgements can be made. In other words they are convinced that the information on the case notes is an accurate rendering of the person who was the subject of that case note. So accurate indeed that modern day psychiatrists can make a judgement about the individual's state of mind and the nature of his/her distress.

To be this accurate it must be the case that the information on the notes is objectively observed and impartially recorded clinical data. If it is so then the language on the case note is a transparent medium through which the subject can be viewed and so the writing clearly represents the individual whose behaviour was being observed. Any hint that the details on the note make up anything less than a clear and untampered with account of the actual doings and sayings of the person who is the subject of the note would discredit the idea that the information contains 'symptoms' which might be interpreted psychiatrically.

There are however, sound reasons for doubting that the information on the case notes can be used as if it was transparent and as if it accurately represented the individuals described on the case note. The most obvious reason for doubting the objectivity of the information is the objection made by linguistic theorists to the idea that language is a clear medium which simply and accurately relays information about the world, an idea that Hayden White calls, 'the illusion on which all of the modern human sciences have been founded . . . that words enjoy a privileged status among the order of things as transparent icons, as value-neutral instruments of representation.'[32] As was suggested in the introductory chapter, such theorists suggest instead that 'language in texts always . . . functions ideationally in the representation of experience and the world.'[33] In other words language is a creative medium, acting to produce new objects (representations and ideas) when describing the world rather than simply reproducing the subjects written about.

Many historians of both medicine and colonialism have been influenced by these linguistic arguments. Those historians who have considered medical knowledge and medical documents[34] in light of such ideas argue along the lines of Ludmilla Jordanova's editorial piece in the *Social History of Medicine*. She concluded that

> it is a mistake to separate the knowledge claims of medicine from its practices, institutions and so on. All are socially fashioned, and so it may ultimately be more helpful to think in terms of mentalities, modes of thought, and medical culture than in terms of 'knowledge', which implies the exclusion of what is inadmissible.[35]

The emphasis then is on the social and cultural nature of medical information rather than on its transparency as a medium for accurately depicting the world. As Jordanova says, medical knowledge is the product of such factors as the mentalities of those writing and the medical culture of the period rather than the result of impartial observation and recording.

In looking at psychiatric records in particular historians have made similar assertions. Jill Matthews argued in her study of female psychiatric patients in twentieth century Australia that the records captured 'the masculine bias of our language and its organisation of reality'[36] rather than produced accurate depictions of the female patients. Cathy Coleborne similarly concluded that the case notes available to her for female patients in nineteenth century Australia were gendered narratives. These told her more about the way in which the male doctors who authored the records thought about and wrote about women than about the individuals who were supposed to be described in the documents. As she says, 'the observations made of the scrutinized patients in the asylum reveal a range of social practices and attitudes towards them.'[37]

Indeed, as was suggested in the introduction it is not only historians of medicine who question the nature of the sources that they work from because of an awareness of the nature of language. Subaltern Studies writers like Shahid Amin and Ranajit Guha have pointed to the ways in which colonial documents create worlds within themselves rather than accurately capturing the reality of the events that they purport to describe. The worlds that are created in these documents are the product of the power relations of the period in which they were written, as Guha says colonial 'texts are not the record of observations uncontaminated by bias, judgement and opinion. On the contrary, they speak of total complicity . . . these documents make no sense except in terms of a code of pacification which, under the Raj, was a complex of coercive intervention by the State and its protégés, the native elite, with arms and words.'[38]

More specifically, writers who have considered colonial psychiatric documents have also emphasised that documents generated by doctors engaged in the administration of those considered insane by the authorities are problematic. Sally Swartz has written about the Valkenberg asylum in turn of the century South Africa.[39] Quite simply, she shows how the information included on case records is not the result of purely scientific observation. Diagnostic patterns reflect professional interests, institutional strategies and medical improvizations. Perhaps most interesting of all is her suggestion that the cultural assumptions of the white doctors about the mentalities of the black patients influenced the diagnostic decisions recorded on case notes. The colonial doctors thought that their black patients were fundamentally different from whites and that their mental experiences would reflect this, and Swartz claims that this was decisive in assessments of the experience of depression among black patients. So, the case notes and asylum records of the Valkenberg Asylum which she studies do not contain information formed by purely medical imperatives. Rather these materials are produced in a political and cultural context, where assumptions and agendas which are the product of power relations in the wider society determine the details included in a medical document.

Once the idea is accepted that language functions ideationally in depiction then the information contained in historical documents is seen as the product of the circumstances in which those documents were written rather than as transparent representations of the apparent subject of the text. In the case of the Valkenberg diagnoses then, as with the diagnoses of Australian women the contemporary psychiatrist attempting retrospective diagnosis would be accepting as medical data information which had been included (and indeed silences which had been imposed) to serve non-scientific, very political purposes. It is therefore necessary to reject the idea that it is possible simply to use historical psychiatric case notes as if they contain objective and accurate observations of the patients that they claim to be records of.

This does not mean that the psychiatric case notes should be adandoned altogether as historical sources. The case notes can be used as products of certain ideas, mentalities and discourses in order to trace those ideas, mentalities and discourses, or as Jonathan

Andrews concluded, 'case notes are innately jaundiced then, in the type of information they record, although this may itself provide quite another eloquent source of insight for the historian, especially into medical discourse and ideologies.'[40] This will be the approach of this chapter then. By analysing the discourses evident in the psychiatric case notes it will be possible to reveal the mentalities, modes of thought and the culture of those who composed the psychiatric case notes of Lucknow.

Discourse analysis: Lucknow's case notes – narratives of colonial fantasy and medical legitimacy

Consider the following case notes:

> Jeeh Singh. m. Dementia. Hindoo. Cultivator. 28. 13 May/ 62.
> Sent from Oonao. Civil Surgeon certifies that he has been insane for 2 months from no apparent cause – at times very violent and disposed to smash everything which comes in his way. Replies very incoherently to questions.
> Shortly after admission he became much quieter- was regularly employed in the garden + improved in health + general appearance. I consider him now quite cured and he is discharged Aug. 5 1862.[41]

> Dabee Singh. Mania. Brahmin. Beggar. 40. 16 April 1861.
> 1861 April. This man was under observation in the Jail for sometime previous to his admission. There he complained that he was kept out of his just and lawful rights + demanded his release. He will eat nothing but sweetmeats. After a time his case was sent in from Hurdui from which it appears that he has been insane for the last three years. That he is not violent but very abusive of all without distinction. He is very much emaciated + suffers from diarrhoea, the effect of the sweetmeats on which alone he subsists.
> June. In the last month has subsisted solely on melons. He eats 12 to 16 per day along with half a pound of chilli. Diarrhoea is less + altho' still there has laid on flesh.
> 1864 This man has been in rude health for the last two years- eats + sleeps well. No difficulty of dieting him. Has regularly worked in the garden – very solicitous for his discharge. Says he has a mother alive in the Hurdui district. Discharged cured 5th Oct 1864.[42]

Both seem to read as narratives of complete mental and physical recovery. Yet these case notes only read as such because of the types of information which have been included on those documents, information which is in fact quite specifically the product of certain modes of writing about the patient. The information on these documents can be separated into two categories. The first is data on the patient's physical condition: Jeeh Singh is 'much improved in health' while Dabee Singh has details of his diet, his emissions and his general physical appearance noted. The second category is not data on the patient's mental condition as might be expected but a record of certain types of behaviour, such as ability to work. The reasons for the decision to include these categories of information need to be explained.

The 'physical': medical legitimacy and the Indian body

The importance of information about the physical condition of the insane patient throughout the period for which case notes are available is emphasized by the examples like that of Bunnoo below:

> Mosst.Bunnoo. Chronic Mania. 35. Moosulman. Beggar. 12th November 1870. Violent.
> 12th Novr 1870. Sent in by the Cantonment Magistrate of Lucknow for re-admission was discharged from asylum on the 5th Novr 1869.
> June 26. 1873. Admitted to hospital for diarrhoea.
> Jan 7. 1874. Bunnoo died this day. She has been insane for about 7 years + in hospital nearly 7 months. She had chronic diarrhoea + became anaemic.[43]

Her entry reads like a chart of a physical demise rather than as a record of mental aberration. The record stresses that she was deemed violent by the Cantonment Magistrate and states simply that she was insane for the best part of seven years by the time she died. Yet the majority of the data concerns her physical condition. The date that her diarrhoea set in, the length of time that she remained afflicted with this bodily condition and the subsequent developments and complications in her physical state were all accorded sufficient significance to enter the case note. This degree of concentration on the physical health of the internee is evident in notes from earlier volumes as well:

> Bholah. m. Mania. 30. Hindoo. Cultr. 24 Jany/ 63
> 1863. Sent in by Deputy Commissioner Roy Bareilly was found wandering about cantonment there – on admission is much attenuated + suffering from dysentery, his intellect appears very much affected but there is also much bodily debility.
> March. This man gradually sunk since his admission – the dysenteric motions improved but he could not eat + the vital powers gradually exhausted. On 23d March, he died.[44]

The only reference to Bholah's mental state on the entire document is a brief mention of the fact that his intellect appeared odd. However, this was not even expanded to the extent that observations on the ways in which this mental state manifested itself were included. The majority of the record is a series of observations on the man's physical condition and afflictions, mentioning his drawn out condition, his weakness and the progress of the disease thought to have had a grip on his body.

A notable feature of the case notes is that death was always recorded when the patient expired in the asylum. Obviously there was a bureaucratic imperative operating as a record of where an individual who was in the system ended up would have been necessary for purposes of internal accounting. However, what is remarkable about this record of death in a document that is ostensibly a record of a sufferer of mental ill health is that information on the causes of death, information that is of its essence a record of the physical causes of a physical demise, was rarely omitted. The above examples each contain details of the circumstances of death and often statements on the case notes were far more explicit. Bhola Dass 'died in hospital from pneumonia'[45] while Goolabdie simply 'died of general debility.'[46] This is similar to Kunsee for who more details are available as she 'died of debility the result of repeated epileptic fits.'[47] Elsewhere Gosalee 'died of chronic diarrhoea,'[48] while a couple of months later Shewrutton 'died of choleric diarrhoea'[49] and a couple of weeks after that Dhavee 'died of chronic dysentery.'[50] The attention to detail in these examples, recording different verdicts on what must after all have been similar ways of dying, is worth noting as are examples such as the following:

> Kem Kurun. 50. Hindu. Labourer. 8 July 1869. Certified by the Magistrate violent.
> 8th July 1869. Sent in by the Depy.Commr.of Oonao in a very weak state.
> 20th July. Died of chronic diarrhoea.[51]

The only opinion arrived at by the medical officer was of this patient's physical condition and the only medical detail recorded was the cause of death. Significantly the column at the top left of the page, where the diagnosed mental condition was usually found, was empty and the only information about the man's behaviour which might be linked to his mental state was supplied by a civil rather than a medical officer. While it can be argued that this patient was alive for less than a fortnight in the custody of the asylum, which was too little time for the medical officer to form an opinion on his mental state, no such explanation can be offered for the example below.

Gokul. Dementia. m. 18. Brahm. Cultivator. 17 Nov/ 64
17th Novr 1864. Sent in by Deputy Commr of Oonao.
29th Septr 1865. Died of chronic dysentery.[52]

While a diagnosis does exist there is no information about the basis for that verdict and the only medical detail in the document of a man who was incarcerated for almost a year because of his supposed mental state was the cause of his physical demise. Quite simply, then, these case notes are dominated by information on the patient's body rather than on his/her mental state. This is reflected in the insistence of the medical officer who compiled the note on entering details surrounding the circumstances of death of the patient.

The most obvious point to make in explaining this focus on the physical is that the asylum superintendent was no specialist in mental illness in this period in British India, the author of the Bengal asylum report of 1877 stating readily that 'few medical officers have had the opportunity of studying insanity.'[53] This comes across in the correspondence between the Government of Madras and the Government of India in 1868/9 in which the arrangements for the new asylum at Madras were debated. The Madras President protested that

> the classification of the insane, the regulation of their common social life under the cottage system, their recreation, their education, their cure, their employment in various descriptions of appropriate labour, all the processes of benevolence and science have to be studied and carried into effect. I do not see how this novel and multifarious duty can be performed here, except by the undivided attention of a medical officer who has bestowed a particular study on the subject.[54]

This was a point that he was reiterating as earlier the Government of India had disagreed with him that the medical officer needed to be 'specially chosen for the duty.'[55] The trouble was that the customary practice in this period was simply to appoint the Civil Surgeon for the town as the superintendent of the local asylum:

> The Medical Officer and Superintendent of the Asylum is the Civil Surgeon of the Station, and has to attend to the Dispensaries, Police and Lock-hospital and other duties pertaining to his appointment.[56]

As such he was unlikely to have any special training in dealing with those deemed to be insane, as was occasionally observed by non-medical officers, 'the Chief Commissioner believes that in India the study and treatment of insanity has not attained the dignity of a *speciality* and that insanes are pretty much left to the care of nature.[57] Indeed there was no reason why the medical officer should have had any special knowledge. For example, the examinations to enter the Indian Medical Service certainly did not require any evidence of work in the field of psycho-medicine: 'the examination covered surgery, medicine (including diseases of women and children), pharmacy, hygiene, anatomy, physiology, botany and zoology.'[58]

In other words, the Civil Surgeon who found himself charged with the superintendence of the local asylum was trained as a physician and a surgeon, not a psychiatrist. His field of expertise was the body and its workings and his day-to-day business in running the dispensaries, lock hospitals and so on would require him to routinely observe, record and treat features of the body. This goes some way to explaining why the asylum case notes are often simply records of physical symptoms. All the superintendent was trained to do was to observe the body and so when confronted in a medical institution with a group of patients he would naturally fall back on what he knew best and most about and get on with the job of observing and recording the bodies of those patients.[59]

There is evidence however that many Indian medical officers took the trouble to read up on mental health theory or at least recalled bits and pieces that they had encountered in medical journals, reference books and so on. So for instance, Dr Wise in the Dacca asylum report of 1872 felt fit to cite 'Sir Charles Hood, in his "Statistics of Insanity" [who] states that in 33.2 per cent of the admissions into Bethlem between 1846–1855, no cause for the madness was ascertained.'[60] He used this evidence to conclude that 'there is little wonder, therefore, that in Bengal we find it extremely difficult to indicate the cause which in each case excites or predisposes to insanity.'[61] The Inspector General of the Indian Medical Department in Bengal quoted Dr Thurnam[62] as 'a writer on the statistics of insanity'[63] in 1872 when discussing rate of recovery amongst asylum patients, and a subsequent Inspector General had evidently consulted the findings of the *Lancet Commission on Lunatic Asylums*. He quoted directly from their report to show that 'only a small proportion can be considered susceptible of cure or radical improvement.'[64] The *Lancet* was not the only source consulted by those involved in asylum administration as Surgeon-Major Payne who was the superintendent of the Dullunda asylum, in discussing the issue of non-restraint in the Report for 1873 decided to 'confine myself to transcribing from the pages of the *British Medical*

Journal (November 11th 1873) a brief summary of advancing opinion in Europe on the question.'[65] In this passage references were made to a number of other sources, the *Edinburgh Medical Journal, Allgemeine Zeits Chrift, Annales Medico-Psychologiques*, so Payne was demonstrating a keen interest in up-to-date discussions of the problems of asylum management.

With this evidence of superintendents in many cases taking a keen interest in the medical theories of the day concerning their charges in the lunatic asylums it is possible to trace discursive circumstances in which the emphasis on physical information in the case notes can be understood. Consider the following account given by Dr Nanney at the Madras asylum in his report for 1878/9:

> In Form 7 are detailed the various causes to which insanity is ascribed. These are divided into physical and moral. It must however be remembered that these divisions are merely arbitrary. The recognition of insanity as a purely physical disease is now gaining ground more surely and it must not be forgotten that the so-called cause is at most an exciting fact, or more probably merely the occasion on which the lurking disorder becomes outwardly manifest.[66]

Dr Nanney was certainly one of the better informed of the superintendents in India. Alongside the above quote he makes reference to such authorities as John Connolly[67] expounding on 'the infirmly sensitive mind bending under the weight of unexpected and sudden trial.'[68] Indeed in other reports[69] he demonstrated himself more than familiar with the nineteenth century's body of thought on mental health issues, mentioning the work of Henry Maudsley,[70] Andrew Duncan,[71] Andrew Wynter[72] and John Charles Bucknill.[73]

What Nanney was insisting on in the above excerpt is an idea that is familiar from studies done of the theories of insanity in Europe in the second half of the nineteenth century. Laurence Ray, in looking at the development of Victorian psychiatry before 1860, concludes that 'insanity was now seen to have a physical basis'[74] and more specifically that 'psychiatric theory regarded insanity as physiologically based in brain pathology.'[75] Andrew Scull agrees with this, pointing to the 'notion that insanity was caused by organic lesions of the brain'[76] and quoting doctors from the time insisting on

> the physiological principle . . . that mental health is dependent upon the due nutrition, stimulation and repose of the brain; that is, upon the conditions of exhaustion and reparation of its nerve substance being maintained in a healthy and regular state; and that mental disease results from the interruption or disturbance of these conditions.[77]

This would certainly explain the details included in the annual reports in India of the appearance of the brain after a post mortem examination. It was believed that if examined thoroughly enough the lesion of the brain, that is the actual alteration of the brain structure, would be visible:

> Luchman an old man, aged about 60 years, who died from epilepsy, had been in the asylum since its establishment in 1864, having been transferred from the old Nagpur Jail. The bones of his skull were much thickened, membranes thickened, and brain atrophied, besides which he had a fatty and enlarged heart.
> Sukaram, in the asylum since 1868, bed ridden for years, remained in hospital from the end of 1879, and died in November from peritonitis. His knees were contracted but there was no other sign of rheumatism. Heart small and pale, but free from adhesion or disease. Brain soft, pale and anæmic, membranes anæmic and not adherent.[78]

Andrew Scull notes a similar dedication to dissecting the brain in England in this period, and points out that even where it was difficult to discern any physiological alteration it was assumed that it was the techniques of post-mortem investigation that were wanting rather than the physicalist assumptions themselves.[79] Again, this adherence to the physicalist theory despite failure to find empirical evidence is a feature of discussions of the issue in India:

> It is true that in cases which in life presented marked symptoms of mental aberration, the nature of a brain organic lesion, if present, eludes us; this should scarcely be subject for wonder while we are as yet unable to tell from looking at a brain the bent of the living man's intellect-cannot distinguish the brain of a great painter or poet from that of a mathematician. The conjecture is a fair one, that alike in both cases there may be differences in mechanism or organization which escape our present means of observation.[80]

German Berrios has shown how this conviction that mental illness had its origins in the physical state of the brain would have resulted in the recording on a case note of all manner of physical information relating, not so much to the brain, as to the rest of the body. He points to

> the analytical and correlational epistemology of the anatomo-clinical view of disease [which] demanded the identification of surface markers, of signs of disease which could represent the anatomical lesion ... The early stages of this process were carefree but soon longitudinal observation, biological markers and statistics introduced a sense of discipline and order.[81]

Indeed, he recently emphasized this, stating that 'a salient difference between pre and post 1900 descriptive psychopathology is that physical (somatic) signs played a far more important role in the former.'[82] He lists such physical symptoms as headaches, tremors, pallor, blushing and changes in bowel or urinary habits and concludes that 'the latter were considered as primary features and as directly related to brain pathology as the typical manifestations of mental disorder.'[83]

Andrew Scull has attempted to relate these theories that mental illness had physical origins and physical symptoms to the power relations of the period. He points to the fact that the medical profession's insistence that mental illness was a matter of physiological disruption served their purposes as an interest group. He identifies three tasks among members of the medical profession in the first half of the nineteenth century:

> Persuading those with power in the political arena of the horrors of the traditional and still flourishing madhouse system and thus of the urgency of reform; establishing asylums run on the new system of moral treatment as the solution to the problem of providing care and treatment for the insane; and reasserting and establishing on a more secure foundation medicine's threatened jurisdiction over madness.[84]

Central to the last part of this project was the development of a fully thought out intellectual rationale for legitimately claiming that madness ought to be the exclusive preserve of those who were medically trained as opposed to being the concern of, for example, those with religious training. Scull directly links the assertion that 'the brain, as a material organ was liable to irritation and inflammation and it was this which produced insanity'[85] to this last part of the project. In other words the physicalist discourses on mental illness were a product of the quest for legitimacy on the part of the medical profession during the nineteenth century.

The nature of the physical information that is included on the case notes from the Lucknow lunatic asylum can be linked to a number of medical discourses then, from discourses of medical legitimacy to the anatomo-clinical gaze. Quite simply, the amount of physical detail on the case notes does not reflect a natural or self-evident way of looking at the mentally ill. Rather, the physical detail is the product of the ways that nineteenth century Western doctors imagined insanity and conceived of illness in general.

Yet a look at the more detailed information about the physical state of the patients suggests that the case notes are not solely linked to these medical discourses. The general observations noted about the cranium of patients in the early 1860s – Chumula for example 'has a low forehead and narrow head'[86] had been replaced by more accurate data by the end of the decade. In the first entry on Kudhlay's record in 1868 is the detail 'circumf of head 20 inches.'[87] Hulwar's entry suggests a determination by the British officer to be thorough in his measurements as 'cir of head $20^5/_8$ in'[88] is scribbled on his case note. The doctor who compiled the document for Dulloo was evidently taking an interest in this part of his job as he did not simply record the measurement but passed the comment that 'his head measures only 20 inches.'[89]

These measurements were of course linked to the phrenological project of recording head size in an attempt to discern correlations between cranial capacity and mental capabilities. This project was part of the general move towards anthropometry in Western culture which had begun in the eighteenth century and which was receiving official endorsement in India by the 1860s with the publication of George Campbell's *The Ethnology of India* in 1865 and the subsequent Ethnological Committee in the Central Provinces of 1866/7.[90] This measuring of bodies grew from what has been called, 'the peculiarly recurring idea that is deeply rooted in Western scientific and popular thought . . . the idea that moral character is rooted in the body'[91] and led to a host of medical and scientific surveys of populations around the world. These were made in the belief that they would enable governments to map out areas where concentrations of bodies considered deviant were believed to signify congregations of problem characters. In India these surveys were collected together in the form of the census, the 'Gazetteers' and the collections of 'Castes and Tribes' records which Rachel Tolen argues, 'were undertaken with the goal of amassing a body of knowledge about the various peoples of India, their customs, and their manners, in order to aid in their efficient administration.'[92] The information about Indian heads on the Lucknow case notes throughout the 1860s is comprehensible then in terms of the very political project of mapping populations which were thought to pose a threat to settled rule by searching for physical correlations to moral or behavioural patterns considered problematic for government.

Yet when remarks on skin colour, 'is of slight build and very dark in complexion, with very bright, restless eyes'[93] or personal hygiene, 'not violent but filthy in his habits,'[94] are included on the case notes it is possible to see how the collection of physical data goes beyond the simple compilation of information for governmental purposes. As David Arnold says, 'over the long period of British rule in India, the accumulation of medical knowledge about the body contributed to the political evolution and ideological articulation of the colonial system.'[95] In other words knowledge of Indian bodies is not just comprehensible in terms of the evolution of systems of effective government, or indeed of nineteenth century medical discourses. The body was a site for the construction of difference and difference lay at the heart of the power relations of the nineteenth century controversies about who was fit to enjoy the privileges of economic, legal and political enfranchisement.[96] People demonstrably different from those who held the power to exclude from the economic and cultural benefits of modernity were considered unfit to be included. As such 'the ideal human body [was] cast implicitly in the image of the robust, European, heterosexual gentleman' resulting in 'the idea that individuals who deviate from that ideal are morally and socially inferior and that their social or moral disruptiveness is always somehow embodied.'[97] The information on Lucknow's case notes on skin colour or the degradation of the patient's approach to his/her own body is not comprehensible in terms of contemporary theories on mental illness. It is comprehensible in terms of what David Arnold called the 'ideological articulation of the colonial system.' In other words these entries on the case notes are not clinical observations which can be understood as uncontaminated scientific data. These entries are located in the project of defining the 'otherness' of those to be excluded from power. In this case it is the colonized Indian who is being demarcated as different from the 'European heterosexual gentleman.'

It would seem then that much of the information on the case notes, data on the patient's body which in so many examples dominates the documents, is the product of discourses linked to the power relations of nineteenth century medical culture, nineteenth century government and nineteenth century colonialism. It would be extremely difficult for the historian to use this data as 'scientific' information which fulfilled the criteria of objectivity sufficiently to qualify for use for diagnosis. The historian however can use it to explore the ways in which bodies were constructed and represented in the nineteenth century from within a variety of political agendas.

Mental illness and recovery: the colonial fantasy of reforming the Indian

Despite the amount of physical information included on the case notes there *are* references to the behavioural state of the patient and the responses of the patient to the therapeutic regimes available in the asylum:

> Heengun Khan. Mania. Mussulman. Cultivator. 26. 30th April 1860.
> Sept, 60. An inhabitant of Moosalbagh. Is said to have been subject to fits of insanity for 12 or 14 years. During intervals has been able to work. Is of a very restless disposition + much taken up with his personal appearance, decorating himself with whatever in the shape of supposed finery falls in his way, not despising as a necklace an old leather Doomchee. Is occasionally violent + continually begs for release. General health and appetite good.
> Oct. 24. For the last month has been generally quiet + well conducted, working hard in the garden + greatly pleased at receiving commendation or trifling rewards. Today became unaccountably violent, had to be confined-blister applied.
> March 1861. For the last three months, there has been a steady improvement in this patient. He takes his meals well + has done bheestie's work very steadily. For the last month his demeanour has so much improved that on his relatives coming to enquire after him I discharged him on the 24th March, cured.[98]

The case note for Heegun Khan reads as a heartening story of improvement as he recovered sufficiently from being fitful and violent to be released to his relatives. Yet look again at the type of information recorded which is in the case note to indicate illness and recovery. Illness is violence and self-absorption. Recovery is obsequious obedience and the desire or ability to work steadily. Pick out the adverbs of illness and recovery: 'unaccountably' as opposed to 'steadily'. The issue to be considered here is whether the privileging of the ability to work and to be governable (because obedient and steady) over the need to be expressive of fluctuating inner desires and feelings (which are unpredictable and sometimes violent) is necessarily a natural correspondence to the state of mentally healthy over mentally ill.

The work of feminist scholars is important here as they are keen to remind that asylum regimes in Europe were not concerned with restoring a natural state of mental health when it came to female patients. Yannick Ripa insists that 'the asylum sought to force women back into the mould from which they had just tried to escape,'[99] and that in France in the nineteenth-century to be cured meant to be submissive. The image of healthy womanhood put forward by the special doctors, those products and exponents of bourgeois society, was of silent women who showed moderation in everything, and who sublimated all their own desires in their role as mothers.[100]

Elaine Showalter finds this to be similar to the experience in England in the same period as 'the ladylike values of silence, decorum, taste, service, piety and gratitude . . . were made an integral part of the program of moral management of women in Victorian asylums.'[101] It was not just in the lunatic asylum that 'recovery' was linked to imposed norms. Joanne Monk examines the Magdalen asylum in Australia which was opened and operated for the reform of 'fallen women' in the 1880s. In it she finds that the regime centred around the performance of laundry duty. Laundry duty was specially chosen as it was seen as an essentially female task and that therefore the correct performance of this task was supposed to signify 'reform', or rather return to the desired norm of domesticated femininity.[102] Reform or recovery in women was very much judged in these institutions not by reference to some natural standard of health and illness but by reference to a standard of behaviour derived from the social and cultural discourses of patriarchy.

With the idea that recovery from mental illness could be a judgement on an individual's compliance with certain prescribed ways of behaving the case note of Heengun Khan included above appears to be rather more than a simple record of the patient's behaviour. Neither was such a case note untypical:

> Ramcharum. Acute mania. 25. Hindoo. Beggar. 11th May 1870. Certified by the Magistrate violent.
> 11th May. Sent in by the Depy.Commr.of Oonao. It appears to be a case of mania from excessive bhung smoking.
> 14th April 1874. For several months Ramchuram has seemed to be in his right mind. He has been useful in helping to cook for the other patients. To be brought before the Committee.
> 7th April 1874. Cured, made over to his friends by order of his friends.[102]

This case note from towards the end of the period for which case notes are available records the direct relationship between the ability to work and the assessment of recovery. The only information included to justify the statement that he seemed to be in his right mind is that he was eventually able to labour and was useful. Indeed the doctor who composed the following example from the second volume of case notes seems to acknowledge that when he had to comment on whether somebody was mentally 'well' he was actually looking for certain characteristics:

> Wazeeran. f. Mania. 28. Mussul. Beggar. 15 Jany/ 63
> 1863. Sent in by City Magistrate found knocking about the City, is very violent and wild in manner and expression.
> 1868 May 5. This woman has been five years in the asylum. She seems to be well, at least she works + does what she is told + gives intelligent answers to questions + is quiet, eats and drinks + sleeps properly.
> She says she is a prostitute + will return to the exercise of her profession if released.
> May 11. Discharged.[104]

He appears to imply, in qualifying his assessment that she was 'well', that the criteria for being judged 'well' were not an esoteric series of standards regarding proper perceptual relations between the inner life and the outer world but were merely the requirements he lists. In other words he is saying that he would not put his name to a judgement that she was absolutely 'well' but rather that she was considered 'well' as she appeared to be socially functional. The criteria for 'socially functional' were productivity, obedience, intelligibility and self-regulation. There were distinct cultural reasons why it was these characteristics which formed those criteria.

Nikolas Rose gives an account of political economy as an understanding of the universe which developed throughout the nineteenth century in Europe, in which it was thought that the economy was a set of natural, self-regulating mechanisms which operated in a benign way to produce a wealthy and well-organised society.[105] It followed therefore that each individual was expected to earn an independent living by participating in a responsible manner in the labour market. As such those who chose not to engage in the economic system, typically those who refused to sell their labour, were condemned as flouting the natural and beneficent mechanisms. Such people became the focus of asylums and workhouses, as a belief in the essential morality of man had encouraged the idea that such people were in need of reform as within them existed the essence of a moral (industrious, compliant, deferential, modest[106]) person which simply needed encouragement.

The characteristics connected with the virtues of work and the ethics of political economy were certainly valued by the British in India by the 1860s, 'the qualities that were most prized were efficiency, practicality, conformity,'[107] as they sought to create, 'a socio-economic environment that rewarded hard work, thriftiness, and a desire to get ahead.'[108] This enthusiasm for political economy and the corresponding enthusiasm for the virtues connected with work explains why the ability to labour in an Indian lunatic patient would have featured so heavily in the case note compiled by a British officer. The culture of political economy dictated that industry was good, indeed natural, so the evidence of a previously disruptive individual beginning to work would have been represented in this cultural frame of references as a 'recovery' of the natural state. Quite simply the case note was a site where the nineteenth century European conviction that the desire to labour was natural and normal was constructed.

Indeed it was within this language of the virtues of work and the ethics of political economy that a discourse of difference was constructed by nineteenth century European men. Nancy Fraser demonstrates how work in the West was one of the key areas in which gender difference was constructed: 'Take the role of the worker. In male dominated, classical, capitalist societies, this role is a masculine role . . . there is a very deep sense in which masculine identity in these societies is bound up with the breadwinner role.'[109] Women's work was constructed as reproduction rather than production and where women were expected to perform productive tasks these tasks were carefully fenced off as different and inferior.

Similarly in the colonies difference was constructed between the Europeans and the locals in terms of their productive capabilities. Racial discourses on the 'lazy native'[100] created images of Africans and Asians in the colonisers' minds as unwilling and inefficient labourers. In India this supposed inability of Indians to work effectively was itself construed by the colonisers as a reflection on Indian society and the Indian psyche. Ronald Inden points out that the Indian mentality was constructed as the opposite of the Western one on the basis of discourses of work and productivity:

> That mind is . . . governed by passions rather than will, pulled this way and that by its desire for glory, opulence, and erotic pleasures or total renunciation rather than prompted to build a prosperous economy and orderly state. The Indian mind is, in other words, devoid of 'higher', that is, scientific rationality.[111]

Crucially, it was exactly this construction which encouraged the British belief that their role in India was necessary: 'It is the supposed absence of these assumed attributes of Western culture – such as advanced rationality, individual discipline, and social habits of obedience – that mark the Indians as childlike creatures in need of paternal oversight.'[112] The British role moreover was often conceived as more than simply 'oversight.' The growing influence of Utilitarian ideas in the British administration of India by the 1860s[113] meant that many colonisers believed that 'it was more important to civilize than subdue'[114] and that many intended that 'the whole of Indian society would undergo a vast transformation, setting it on a rapid advance up the scale of civilization.'[115] In other words the British fantasised that they would transform India from 'uncivilized', that is irrational and unproductive to 'civilized', that is ordered, industrious and regular. Mukhsoodally Khan was thus transformed according to his case note:

> Mukhsoodally Khan. m. amentia. mussul. service. 25. 8 June/ 61
> 1861 June. This man was formerly a sowar in the 1st Regt. of Hodson's Horse at Fyzabad. Was admitted into Regl.Hospital on 14th May on account of mania – cause not apparent – He was noisy, violent + abusive, bit himself on legs + arms + required the constant supervision of attendance to prevent his escaping or injuring himself. Subsequently he had an attack of fever. On admission he was very excitable and talked very unnaturally and abusively.
> 1862 Feb. In several months past this man has improved in health, has been quiet + well conducted and assisted in the garden. He is stout + strong. All bodily functions properly performed + he does not appear to be labouring under any delusion. His relatives are anxious to remove him + I therefore, as he has been well for months, discharge him cured.[116]

Violent, irrational ('talked very unnaturally') and unpredictable ('cause not apparent') he was represented as becoming regulated ('all bodily functions properly performed'), respectful and a good worker. His case note is a narrative of the fantasy of the colonial project where the Indian Other of the rational and productive European is civilized, that is made rational and productive, through contact with the benign British institution. A glance at Heengun Khan's case note at the beginning of this section suggests that Muksoodally Khan's case note is not unique in reading as such a narrative. Heengun Khan was constructed as narcissisitic and violent at the outset of the case note but by the end was represented as self-disciplined and productive after a spell under British control.

The information on the behaviour of the patients included on the document is not the result of impassive and objective surveillance of the individual in question. That information is instead the product of the imaginings and expectations of a British medical officer during the period of 'high colonialism'. The information on work, violence and self-discipline acts to create on the case note a world where work is natural and normal, where Indians are unproductive and irrational and where contact with the British regime is so beneficial and effective that Indians become 'civilized.' Quite simply, the case notes are sites where the colonisers constructed India and Indians as the Other of the colonisers and where they represented colonialism as an effective system of rendering useful those they considered unproductive and irrational.

Conclusion

> Patient records are surviving artefacts of the interaction between physicians and their patients in which individual personality, cultural assumptions, social status, bureaucratic expediency, and the reality of power relationships are expressed.[117]

The case notes from the Lucknow asylum read less as a series of objective observations of naturally occurring conditions and more as a collection of statements which construct ideals of social and moral fitness, which reflect culturally specific modes of seeing and which legitimize colonial rule. The discourses traced here, of the significance of the Other's body, of the possibility of reforming the Indian mentality, of the medical gaze, are all linked to power relations in the period, to the fantasies and projects of European bourgeois masculinity, to the colonial order, to the rise of the medical profession and so on. By tracing them it is possible to identify a number of the ways that the British saw themselves and Indians in the context of late nineteenth century colonial India.

For this reason the historian may legitimately use sources like the asylum records of British India to trace the relationship between power and knowledge but the researcher must be wary of looking at the records in the hope of using them to explore the epidemiology of the past. One reason for such wariness is the doubts about the accuracy and consistency of much of the information on the case notes. The more important reason however is that the records of the lunatic asylum provide compelling evidence of power relations in colonial India as the details of supposedly scientific documents like a psychiatric case note turn out to be a series of representations and judgements of the Indian. They fail therefore to provide much evidence of the mental states of the Indians of which they are supposed to be a record. Their value as a historical source lies in what they can tell the historian about the ways that the colonial imaginations looked at and constructed Indians. The irony then is that in acting as records of the ways that the British saw and represented India and Indians, the psychiatric case notes of the Indian patients offer little by way of insight into Indian mental states but plenty by way of evidence of British ones.

2

'The Lunatic Asylums of India are Filled with Ganja Smokers': Asylum Knowledge as Colonial Knowledge

David Arnold concluded in an article dealing with the prisons of the British colonial system in India:

> I would argue that medical research and administration in Indian prisons had an exceptional role not only in medical research but also in creating a colonial discourse about Indian society and the Indian body.[1]

He was making the point that the prison was a site, one of the few such sites, where the British had unlimited access to the Indian body. As such, the information gathered there was privileged as rare data and came to be regarded as representative of all of India and of all Indians rather than just of those who ended up within the prison walls.

This chapter will consider the asylum in a similar way, and demonstrate how the information generated at the asylum came to assume importance beyond the confines of the superintendent's office. Indeed, the chapter will follow on from the previous chapter in showing how the ways of seeing Indians and India of the superintendents at the asylums generated images and fantasy social threats which came to concern colonial government in general and indeed even troubled parliamentary government in London.

Parliament and cannabis

Cannabis entered British political discourse in 1891 when Mark Stewart was moved to ask the Under-Secretary of State for India whether his attention has been called to the statement in the *Allahabad Pioneer* of the 10th May last that ganja 'which is grown, sold and excised under much the same conditions as opium', is far more harmful than opium, and that 'the lunatic asylums of India are filled with ganja smokers.'[2]

Yet when Mark Stewart first asked this there was certainly no perceived problem of domestic cannabis abuse in the United Kingdom. Rather opium and alcohol use among the working classes was becoming a concern.[3] Indeed cannabis was little used in Victorian Britain and rarely discussed outside medical and intellectual circles. It was in India and in the colonial administration that there first developed a concern about the social implications of people using preparations of hemp. As early as 1871 the Government of India had contacted British civil officers, doctors and soldiers throughout South Asia for information on the issue of whether 'the abuse of ganja produces insanity and other dangerous effects.'[4]

The report which gathered together their replies[5] was forwarded to Britain in 1892 as a response to Mark Stewart's question and was lodged in the House of Commons library by William Caine MP. It was Caine who asked the subsequent question in the House of Commons in March 1893 which was to lead to the establishment of the Indian Hemp Drugs Commission (IHDC) in April of that year. This Parliamentary Commission was charged with going to India in order to 'inquire into the cultivation of the hemp plant in Bengal, the preparation of drugs from it, the trade in these drugs, the effect of their consumption upon the social and moral condition of the people, and the desirability of prohibiting the growth and the sale of ganja and allied drugs.'[6] It received information from over 1000 witnesses across India between October 1893 and April 1894 and reported back to Parliament later that year.

The earliest discussions of cannabis preparations in British political discourse appear then to have been reliant for information and for opinion on the experiences of British government in India. This was no coincidence as the concerns of administrators in India about cannabis had in fact generated these discussions in Britain.

India and images of cannabis

In relying on India for information about hemp preparations Mark Stewart, William Caine and the British government were very much in keeping with patterns established earlier in the nineteenth century. What discussion there was in Britain of cannabis preparations had come from Indian examples and experiences since at least the 1820s. In 1826 in London Whitelaw Ainslie published the first book length account of Indian medicines of the British colonial period. He observed of ganja that, 'the leaves of the hemp in India, are frequently added to tobacco and smoked to increase its intoxicating power; they are also sometimes prescribed in cases of diarrhoea; and in conjunction with turmeric onions, and warm ginglie oil, are made into an unction for painful, protruded piles.'[7]

Apparently then, while intoxicating, hemp was also considered the source of potentially valuable medicine. This is a theme which subsequent British writers developed. W.B. O'Shaughnessy conducted a number of experiments in Calcutta with hemp derivatives in the 1830s. The results were subsequently published in the *Transactions of the Medical and Physical Society of Bengal*.[8] His observation of animal reactions to hemp preparations, for example a 'middling-sized dog' whose 'face assumed a look of utter helpless drunkenness',[9] gave him an awareness of the stupefying effects of the drug. However, the potential as a medicine in some of the other effects, 'of stimulating the digestive organs, exciting the cerebral system [and] in allaying pain' was such that experiment on humans was decided upon. Rheumatism, Hydrophobia, Cholera, Tetanus and 'infantile convulsions' were all treated successfully with various hemp concoctions and O'Shaughnessy concluded that 'in Hemp the profession has gained an anti-convulsive remedy of the greatest value.'[10] O'Shaughnessy's work came to be used as a standard text for those writing on hemp derivatives throughout the nineteenth century. The *Encyclopaedia Britannica* for example quoted his work as a source in its entry on hemp alongside 'Dr Royle's Illustrations of the Botany of the Himalayan Mountains' in 1856.[11]

Information available in the UK in the first half of the nineteenth century about cannabis came from India and generally reflected the curiosity of the British in India about the possible uses of preparations of the hemp plant as a medicine. As the century progressed however attitudes in India towards hemp began to darken and, as mentioned above, by 1871 the Government of India decided to conduct a survey of its officers on the subject. It stated in its circular that

It has been frequently alleged that the abuse of ganja produces insanity and other dangerous effects.

The information available in support of these allegations is avowedly imperfect, and it does not appear that the attention of the officers in charge of lunatic asylums has been systematically directed to ascertain the extent to which the use of the drug produces insanity.

But as it is desirable to make a complete and careful enquiry into the matter, the Governor-General in Council requests that Madras, Bombay etc. will be so good as to cause such investigations as are feasible to be carried out in regard to the effects of the use or abuse of the several preparations of hemp. The inquiry should not be simply medical but should include the alleged influence of ganja and bhang in exciting to violent crime.[12]

The responses to the inquiry showed that there was in many parts of India a mistrust of cannabis preparations and of those who used them. 'Hushiarpur says that in March 1864 the Nehung Sikh who killed the Reverend Mr Janviers (missionary) was a known bhang drinker'[13] asserted the Punjab authorities, while Hyderabad forwarded the opinion that 'it is generally said, and I believe with much truth, that when a man "runs amuck" or a female commits "suttee" that before committing the act they are intoxicated by the use of hemp in some form or other.'[14] Those in Berar were afraid that, 'Bhang is also taken by immoral people as an 'aphrodisiac' as tending to excite the sexual passions. Preparations of hemp are also much used by women for the purpose of procuring abortion,'[15] while an old medical officer serving in Burma was able to assert that 'most of the acts of Mutiny of 1857 were undertaken under the influence of bhang, charas or ganja.'[16]

By 1885 these negative associations were being repeated in medical journals where earlier in the century there had been scientific debate about cannabis. The *Indian Medical Gazette* published the following piece:

ASSAULTS BY GANJA SMOKERS

Murderous assaults by individuals under the influence of Indian hemp have been somewhat frequent of late in Bombay. At the Bombay Police Court, towards the end of May last, two cases of this nature came up for trial . . . In the one case the prisoner Khuda Baksh, without provocation struck with his fists a Parsee child aged 2 1/2 years which was being carried along the street by an older girl. He thereafterwards seized the child by the legs and dashed its head on the ground. He was then seized by the passers by and on being brought before the Magistrate pleaded guilty saying that he at the time was under the influence of ganja, and did not know what he was doing. As the child recovered from the concussion of the brain the man was only sentenced to six months vigorous imprisonment. In the second case a Moghul, named Syed Hossein Ali Khan, while under the influence of ganja was walking in the street with an open knife in his hand when he made a thrust at another Moghul with his knife. The attacked individual by stepping backwards received only a comparatively superficial wound over the stomach. The assailant then fled through the bazaar like a maniac brandishing the knife and threatening every one in his neighbourhood. He was seized with much difficulty and was sentenced to six months rigorous imprisonment. A very large number of inhabitants of this country are addicted to this form of intoxication and the present low price of the drug allows of its being too readily procurable so that further restrictions on its sale are certainly called for in order to lessen this source of bodily danger to which the public are constantly exposed.[17]

Evidence from British journals shows that the medical press was a means by which information about cannabis was fed from India back to the UK. *The Lancet* in 1880 published a report which reflected the increasingly negative approach to cannabis use and cannabis users in India. It directly linked madness, violence and death with the use of hemp preparations:

POISONING BY INDIAN HEMP: AUTOPSY

The *Indian Medical Gazette* reports a case of death resulting from Indian hemp, some preparation of which the deceased had been accustomed to smoke for many years. After so indulging he generally became insensible or stupid. He was delirious for a fortnight before his death. On the day on which he died he tried to hammer a nail into his temple, and then expired suddenly . . . beneath the dura mater blood was found effused over the whole upper surface of right brain and over the frontal lobe of left brain. A large clot was found in the right middle fossa of skull; this extended across the crux and pons . . .[18]

In summary then, cannabis use by 1871/3 was associated by colonial officials with infanticide, immorality, suicide, the murder of Christians, and even the revolt against British authority of 1857. The cannabis user was identified as a human type, seen as unpredictable, violent and the proper subject of such Western investigative techniques as the post-mortem. As India had throughout the nineteenth century been the source of information about hemp preparations these attitudes had begun to filter back into Britain by the 1880s. As such it comes as no surprise to discover that when in the 1890s Mark Stewart raised the issue of cannabis in Parliament he took his examples from India, in this case from the newspaper the *Allahabad Pioneer*. Indeed, it is also possible to see why when he did take information from India this information was damning.

Yet it must be noted that many of the responses to the 1871 inquiry reveal that not all British administrators in India had negative opinions of cannabis or of cannabis users. It appears that many believed, as did those in the Central Provinces,

> and apparently not without great show of reason, that persons whose employment subjects them to great exertions and fatigues, such as palki-bearers &c., are solely enabled to perform the wonderful feats that they not unfrequently do, by being supported and rendered insensible to fatigue by ganja; and the use of ganja leaves in them no after effect of an injurious kind.[19]

There were then officers who had views of the hemp user which were opposed to those which regarded him as violent or lunatic. It seems that there were also those who were oblivious to the issue, unable to offer an opinion one way or the other on cannabis use and its effects. For example in the summary of reports in Bombay it was noted that 'most of the Superintendents of Jails write to say they have no experience as to the extent the abuse of ganja proves an incentive to crime, and few of them seem to have had their attention drawn to the subject.'[20]

There appears to be evidence then of a lack of consensus among British administrators in India on the subject of cannabis and cannabis use in the 1870s. Yet the resolution of the GOI at the end of the cannabis inquiry begun in 1871 prohibited the cultivation and consumption of ganja in Burma and urged other areas of India to 'discourage the consumption of ganja and bhang by placing restrictions on their cultivation, preparation and retail, and imposing on their use as high a rate of duty as can be levied without inducing illicit practices.'[21] In other words it dismissed dissenting voices and opted for a policy which betrayed a distrust of cannabis preparations. Similarly it was the negative opinions of cannabis and cannabis use which made their way from India to Parliament in the 1890s as Mark Stewart and William Caine based their questions on them. The nature of these negative opinions and the process by which they came to dominate the discussion of hemp preparations in India in the 1870s and by which they came to trouble Parliament in the 1890s will be explored in the rest of this article. In tracing this process the article will explore the ways in which the fancies of asylum administrators became a matter of enquiry in the House of Commons.

Cannabis and the asylums of India

The constant reference to the lunatic asylums of British India in discussions of cannabis and cannabis users is the first clue in tracing the origins of those discussions. Mark Stewart of course specifically referred to the asylums in his question to Parliament and there were those who in the 1870s were invoking them as the source of evidence in support of their arguments. 'The Commissioner has always looked on a ganja-smoker and a bad character as synonymous, and has, in his connection with lunatic asylums in different parts of Bengal, observed that in a large number of cases insanity has been induced by excessive ganja-smoking.'[22] Indeed the GOI Resolution at the conclusion of the 1871 inquiry also extensively quoted evidence from asylums throughout India in support of its conclusions. Asylums in the Central Provinces, Mysore, the Punjab and Bengal are all mentioned in the Resolution and a reproduction of the table of Dr Penny at the Delhi institution is included along with excerpts of his conclusions. 'Of 317 lunatics received into the Nagpur Asylum since 1864, there were 61 in whom insanity had been occasioned by an immoderate use of ganja ... From this result it is inferred that excess in ganja-smoking does produce an insanity which is transient.'[23]

The asylum was important as it was the site of what will be called here the categorization and the enumeration of cannabis use as a social problem. Arjun Appadurai has identified these two stages by which official colonial knowledge was generated.[24] His case study examines the ways in which 'caste' became a means of understanding Indian society for the British administrators of India in the nineteenth century. Anthropological work of eighteenth and early nineteenth century colonizers emphasized the importance of caste categories as the key for the British to mapping Indian society. It was only when the census provided a means of counting people within the categories of the caste system that that knowledge system became the predominant mode of conceiving of Indian society. The census was so important as 'numbers were a critical part of the discourse of the colonial state, because the metropolitan interlocutors of the colonial state had come to depend on numerical data, however dubious their accuracy and relevance, for major social or resource-related policy initiatives.'[25]

The two separate stages, categorization and enumeration, by which cannabis use became conceived of as a social problem for the British will be considered at the asylum.

The asylum and categorization

There were two stages by which cannabis use and cannabis users became categorized as a social problem in the asylums of colonial India. First, medical officers at the asylums came to believe that cannabis use was linked to insanity and violence in Indians. Second, the officers used the asylum as a site where they could observe cannabis users and establish the distinguishing signs which marked them off as a distinct human type to be watched out for because of their dangerous potential.

The British superintendents of the asylums came to believe that cannabis was linked to insanity and violence as they were told by the Indian policemen who had picked the inmates up that many of the people that they brought to the asylum were there because of excessive use of hemp. Perhaps more importantly the doctors who received this police information had reasons not to dismiss this information and to note it in their records.

Consider the opinion of the Dr Simpson in the asylums report for Bengal in 1874: 'Among the pauper class information as to the cause, unless the case be that of a known ganja-smoker, is often not procurable; and as the formal statement of the cases includes a direct question, an imaginary cause is entered.'[26] He goes on to point out that 'judging from the style of the answers furnished by the police in the descriptive rolls, it would appear that if the man be a ganjah-smoker the drug is invariably put down by them as the cause of insanity.'[27] What he is describing is a process in which the police, who needed to come up with a cause of insanity to complete the forms correctly, often could find no evidence of what had disrupted the behaviour of the individual that they wished to incarcerate. This meant that they would have to make one up, and in such a situation 'ganjah-smoking' was a convenient and accepted way of filling the form up and one that was likely to be believed.[28]

'Ganjah-smoking' as cause of insanity on the form was likely to be accepted by the medical officers at the asylums despite the dubious ways in which the police arrived at that judgement. The first reason for this was that many in India shared the opinion of the Commissioner of Sitapur that preparations of hemp, by virtue of their intoxicating properties, were comparable to alcohol and opium and were therefore an irredeemable evil likely to lead to mental problems:

In his own court Commissioner has seen more than one instance in which the criminal pleaded, in excuse or explanation of violence or murder, that the crime was committed when under the influence of bhang; and there is in his mind no doubt that the use of the drug operates much as intoxicating liquors do in England, by stimulating the passions and weakening the power of self-control.[29]

There was also a more specific reason why this credence was given. Throughout the nineteenth century medical men in Europe were struggling to assert their authority over the psyche. In other words doctors needed to prove that the brain and its workings were properly their concern and not the concern of other professional groups like the clergy who could claim specialist knowledge of the routes to psychological well-being. As such 'ascribing aetiologies was important because it gave a sense, often illusory, of having the means to predict, prevent and control the spread of mental disorder.'[30] Indeed the emphasis on an external stimulant as a cause of insanity corresponded neatly with contemporary medical theories that 'the brain, as a material organ was liable to irritation and inflammation and it was this which produced insanity,'[31] theories which insisted upon the physiological basis of mental illness in order to assert the jurisdiction of medical men over insanity. Blaming hemp was a simple and plausible way of ascribing the aetiology of mental disease in India which thereby reinforced the medical officer's claim that he knew what he was talking about.

Medical officers therefore became convinced that they were observing many hemp users at the asylums. In fact what they observed were individuals who had only come to their attention in the first place as their behaviour was so visibly disordered or disruptive that the police had felt it necessary to intervene and send them to an asylum. This person's behaviour had been ascribed to use of cannabis preparations, often by Indian policemen who had very little evidence that this was indeed the case. Individual case notes therefore came to read as following:

Bhugwan Dass. Mania acute. 26. Hindoo. labour. 23 Feby/ 69. Certified by Magistrate violent
28 Feb 1869. Probably from bhung. He is very troublesome + destructive. Sent in by City Magistrate of Lucknow.
3rd May. Made over to his friends by order of the committee.[32]

As this is the entire case note it seems that all the information available for Bhugwan Dass is that he was destructive and that this was thought to have been the result of the man's use of a preparation of hemp. The implication of the qualification 'probably' suggests that the medical officer had no direct evidence that hemp was the cause of the man's behaviour yet he was happy to record the conjecture. The case note for Allya Khan reads in a similar way:

> Allya Khan. M. Mania. 30. Mussulman. Coolie. 17th Jany/ 63.
> 1863. Sent in by City Magistrate found wandering about Bazar in City is an inhabitant of Lucknow . . . apparently had been smoking and using some drugs to excess was violent on admission.
> Discharged much improved. Made over to his friends.
> June 10th. Readmitted having thrown himself down a well. Is worse than ever.[33]

Again, there is only a tenuous connection with cannabis preparations yet the case note acts as a site where an example of madness through use of hemp narcotics is established. The point is that the only contact that medical officers at the asylums had with those that they thought to be users of hemp preparations was with people who they perceived to be insane and who they saw to be unpredictable and violent. However, from these individual instances which were considered by the doctors at the asylums to be examples of Indian bodies interacting with hemp preparations were built grand generalizations:

> Each and all of these forms of Indian hemp act on the nervous system, exercising a peculiar influence over the brain and spinal chord, and their nerves. They also paralyze the sympathetic nervous system, as shown in the arrest of the secretion of the salivary glands . . . There is a state of brain produced by over-indulgence in bhang or charas, which corresponds to delirium tremens; sudden suspension of its use causing a state of most violent excitement. The patient talks incessantly; pelts those about him with bricks or stones; bites and tears his clothes; and it would be dangerous to approach him . . . He may die from exhaustion of the brain, or stoppage of the heart's action from paralysis of the sympathetic, or he may gradually recover.[34]

This report is included in the replies of the Bengal Government to the inquiry of 1871 and is an extract from Dr Penny's report on the Patna asylum. Despite the fact that the sample from which he has formed his opinions is simply those he has watched in the asylum, he generalizes or universalizes his conclusions and talks of 'the brain' or 'the nervous system' rather than specific brains or individual nervous systems. Having universalized his subject he moves on to the effects of hemp and then on to the behaviour of 'the patient' rather than 'a patient', who is violent and dangerous, and indeed liable to sudden death.

This is the crucial step between observing individuals at the asylum and establishing cannabis use and cannabis users as a social problem in colonial discourse. The specific becomes the universal, in other words the disordered individual whose odd behaviour has been linked at the asylum with hemp use becomes representative of all hemp users. This is because he is the only point of access that the British, and especially those with the medical training to claim scientific authority for their opinions, have to Indian people thought to use hemp. The ordinary Indian who while going about his business enjoys a smoke or a drink of some hemp preparation will never come to the attention of the British and be examined or recorded by them. Rather it is the disordered individual available to the medical gaze in the institutional setting of the asylum and produced on the case note as a hemp user that represents the sole access that the British have to Indians thought to use hemp. Thus their violence, weakness or disruption comes to be regarded as typical of people who use hemp.

The asylum then was the site where the link between the hemp preparations, the hemp user, madness and violence was established in the imagination of many medical officers in India. It was also the site which afforded the means of identifying the users considered so prone to violence and madness. In other words, the category of the hemp user was established not just through identifying the characteristic behaviour that might be expected of such a human type but also through the identification of the physical characteristics of that type.

The search for physical manifestations of mental type is familiar from various accounts of nineteenth century medical research. Jan Goldstein in his study of French psychiatry conjures up the image of the '"sharp-eyed" psychiatrist, whose classification of diseases by their visible signs is his stock in trade and his claim to power.'[35] He goes on to mention the boon photography gave in the compilation of 'a giant and often grotesque archive of the iconography of nervous illness, extending . . . to bodily postures as well as to facial expressions.'[36]

The best known example of attempts to establish a system of irrefutable physical signifiers of moral and mental capacities and processes is the project of phrenology. The phrenologist believed that the careful classification of head size, volume and shape would lead to an understanding of brain size and characteristics. This understanding it was felt would correlate with the nature of the person. Rather than rely on the impressions one had of an individual, the scientific analysis of the head would give the observer the opportunity to scientifically determine the character of the individual. As De Giustino points out in his study of British phrenology there thus grew up a generation of 'men who believed in the shape of the head as an index to character,'[37] where leading exponents of the 'science' 'boasted of phrenology as the useful and long-awaited instrument for separating good men from bad.'[38] The desire in India to observe physical signifiers believed to be important in divining mental state or capacity is shown in the case notes by the occasional note of a phrenological nature.[39] Although never systematic, different doctors at different times did record information on cranial measurements. In 1860 the doctor in charge in Lucknow records that Chumula, 'a stout boy . . . has a low forehead and narrow head,'[40] while in 1868 the note 'circum. of head 20 inches' follows the information that Kudhlay was 'V.violent + dirty. To be kept under strict observation. Destroyed two blankets.'[41]

Various accounts show that doctors used the asylum in colonial India as a site to observe the body of the hemp user, and to build up a picture in their own minds of the physical features by which a user could be recognized. Dr Penny, who was mentioned earlier on, took care to set out a description of the physical characteristics of hemp users; 'Old Bhang drinkers, charas and ganja-smokers and majum-eaters are, as a rule, emaciated. They lose vital energy, become impotent, forgetful, weak-minded and melancholy . . . again charas-smokers are often asthmatic.'[42] The information contained in the Patna superintendent's report for 1868 is even more direct. Consider the page reproduced from the report (Figure 2.1).[43]

Surgeon Hutchinson went as far as to graphically represent the finger of a 'confirmed gunjah-smoker' in order to offer an easy means of identifying such a figure. The language he uses confirms his project in producing the drawing, he is hoping to pass on physical information which will certainly 'betray the habitué' and ultimately 'reveal him'. Such language suggests that he believes hemp users to be surreptitious and that there is a need to establish foolproof ways of uncovering them. He sees the corn as a form of stigmata, an irrefutable sign which when read informs the observer that the man is a hemp user and is therefore under suspicion of being mad, violent, self-destructive and so on. He supplies additional helpful informa-

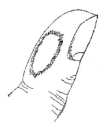

Figure 2.1 The Ganja-corn

Source: *Asylums in Bengal for the Year 1868*, p. 37.

tion, noting such things as, 'a peculiar leery look which, when once seen is unmistakable', and pointing out that, 'a confirmed gunjah smoker has frequently dark, purple lips', but whatever the difficulties of these indicators he assures the reader that, 'the corn and inhalation will always reveal him'. He is plainly trying to record ways in which the hemp user might be recognized physically and in the process creates an image to be attached to a human type or category. The asylum then was the site where the hemp user of the colonial imagination was figuratively 'given flesh.'

To summarize then, information supplied to the superintendents at the asylums linked the use of a variety of hemp preparations to insanity and to unpredictable and violent behaviour. Despite the often dubious nature of this information, many of the superintendents believed it as it corresponded with their general misgivings about intoxicants like opium and alcohol and fitted in with their beliefs about the physiological origin of madness. As the only hemp users that were encountered by these superintendents were those who were under their charge at the asylum because of their disordered or violent behaviour, those medical officers based their opinions of all in India who used cannabis substances on that small and un-representative sample. As these people at the asylum were often violent or unpredictable and were taken to be typical of all hemp users the assumption made was that all hemp users had the poten-tial to be dangerous because of their use of cannabis substances. As such those at the asylum were observed closely for distinguishing marks which they all had in common, marks by which the danger-ous human type identified as the hemp user by medical officers could be detected before individuals became violent or mad. Through this process at the asylum use of cannabis substances among the

Indian population became crystallized as a category of social problem by the colonial authorities through the invention of the hemp user as a dangerous human type.

The asylum and enumeration

Yet the stage of categorization, that is the observation of characteristics and the assignment of type, is only one part of the process that Appadurai says is crucial to the production of official knowledge. As already mentioned Appadurai identified enumeration as the second crucial stage of the process of producing colonial knowledge as 'numerical glosses constituted a kind of meta-language for colonial bureaucratic discourse within which more exotic understandings could be packaged.'[44] The final part of this chapter looks at the asylum as the site of the statistical articulation of hemp users as a social problem and the way that these statistics 'however dubious their accuracy and relevance' allowed the hemp user to enter the discourse of colonial government.

In amongst the range of data collected at the asylum and compiled in the asylum statistics was information on 'cause of insanity of those admitted.' In Bengal for example, where the statistics collected were most complex, there were 21 possible causes mooted in the various asylums in 1870 and 22 by 1875. They were divided into physical causes and moral causes. Amongst the physical were such factors as 'epilepsy' or 'miscarriage' and among the moral 'grief' or 'family quarrel'. Gunjah was always the most occupied category of cause in the known physical causes column in India throughout the 1860s and 1870s.

The passing of comment on the preponderance of hemp narcotics in the statistical table on causes became a routine part of the statement of superintendents. For example, the superintendent of Dullunda commented in 1867 that 'among the causes of admissions, there appear nothing of novelty or special interest. The fact which each succeeding year brings prominently forward, of the prevalence of ganja smoking as a fertile source of insanity is as prominent as ever in the records of 1867.'[45] In 1871 Surgeon Cutcliffe pointed out in his report on the asylum at Dacca that 'Table no. 4 shows the causes to which the insanity of the patients has been attributed. 33 per cent of all the cases are attributed to gunja smoking and 7.18 to spirit drinking.'[46] In 1875 the officer in charge of the asylum in Cuttack pointed out that 'Ganja is reputed as the cause of the majority of the admissions and nearly half of the admissions during the past ten years into this asylum are attributed to its abuse.'[47] Throughout the 1860s and 1870s it was a routine statistical conclusion in the asylums of colonial India that cannabis preparations were responsible in the majority of cases where the cause of insanity was recorded.

Almost as routine was the casting of doubt about the reliability of such statistical conclusions. In 1871 a superintendent voiced his concern that 'causation is, as usual, very unsatisfactorily noted among the admissions. Antecedent information is commonly difficult to procure. Intemperance is an assigned cause in 9 cases, but with one or two exceptions I doubt whether it can be regarded as in any sense a true cause in this number.'[48]

Surgeon Wise admitted in 1872 that

> an attempt has been made this year to distinguish between those cases of insanity clearly due to ganjah-smoking and those in which the use of ganjah has only been occasional, and therefore insufficient to excite insanity. The attempt has not been successful. For want of any other reason, it has been necessary to enter under the heading of ganja several who were merely reported to have indulged in its use.[49]

Dr Simpson, already mentioned for his misgivings about the nature of police information, was content to base an opinion on this information despite his doubts: 'Judging from the style of the answers furnished by the police in the descriptive rolls, it would appear that if the man be a ganjah-smoker the drug is invariably put down by them as the cause of insanity. However this may be, the figures in Table no. 7 impress one with the conviction that ganjah, bhang and alcohol have more to do with the peopling of our asylums than all other cases put together.'[50]

The concern with the accuracy of the statistics was not just restricted to medical officers in Bengal. The medical officer at the Delhi asylum pointed out that, 'I know the difficulties of obtaining information when perhaps the constable who seizes [or] the Thannadar or Deputy Inspector who receives the charge, is himself wanting intelligence.'[51] As late as 1880 Dr Rice at Jubbulpore was still concerned to establish that

> the determination of causes of insanity is of considerably greater difficulty than the classification of the variety. Only too often it is impossible to procure any previous history of the patient. Native relatives (even if any exist and are willing to do so) are not skillful in depicting those

traits of character previous to his seizure which might tend to show
what led to his becoming insane: but too often the man has no known
relatives, and 'shots' are made by the neighbours as to the cause of his
madness.[52]

It is crucial to note though that despite the constant concern
over the relevance and accuracy of the information and of the statistics they were still registered by the non-medical officers reading
the reports and policy was generated on the basis of those numbers. In the report for 1873 for example Surgeon-Major Cayley made
it clear that 'I fear that not much reliance can be placed on the
alleged causes of insanity . . . it is difficult to ascertain if ganja was
the actual cause in so many cases.'[53] However the Judicial Department resolution, written by a civil officer in the Judicial Department
upon receipt of the report, ignored Cayley's misgivings about the
reliability of the figures. It confidently stated that 'there is little
calling for remark on the present report on the types of insanity or
its causes. Of the exciting causes of insanity, ganjah-smoking is
still shown in the returns for the whole of the Lower Provinces as
one of the most frequent; and it is observable that in many cases
of re-admission the patients are said to have been confirmed smokers of the drug.' On the basis of this observation of the statistics
the Judicial Department's resolution recorded that 'the Lieutenant-
Governor is giving special attention to the best means for further
augmenting the check (which has been imposed of late years apparently with some success) on the consumption of this most
deleterious drug.'[54] In other words the statistics of the asylums were
directly responsible for governmental decisions about cannabis use
and cannabis users. It did not matter that medical officers responsible for those statistics actually reported that there were problems
with understanding exactly what they signified. As described by
Appadurai, numerical data, however dubious their accuracy and
relevance, were the meta-language of colonial government. Once
statistics existed, that which they described existed in the minds of
colonial administrators who responded with social policy initiatives.
    Indeed the importance of the statistics generated in the asylums
in securing the entry of the hemp user into the discourse of colonial government is underlined in looking in more detail at the
significance attached to those statistics in the inquiry of 1871. The
statistics produced in the medical institutions were often central to
the replies of non-medical government officers to the GOI inquiry.

The reply from the office of the Chief Commissioner to the Central Provinces includes the information that

> Dr Beatson, Civil Surgeon Nagpur and superintendent of the asylum reports that out of 317 lunatics received into the asylum since 1864, there were 61 in whom insanity had been occasioned by an immoderate indulgence in ganja. Of these 61, 10 have died, 28 have been discharged cured and 23 remain uncured. He therefore concludes that excess in ganja smoking does produce an insanity which is transient if the habit is relinquished but otherwise permanent.[55]

Similarly, the reply from Mysore quotes the figures of the asylum superintendent Dr Ranking which show 'that out of a total of 250 admissions in the lunatic asylum in Bangalore during the past five years the use of ganja is assigned as the cause of insanity in 82 cases, but 64 persons of the number so affected subsequently recovered their reason, and were discharged.'[56] The whole report of Dr Penny at the Delhi asylum is reproduced in the reply of the Punjab and a statistical table tracing the percentages of the total treated for hemp related mental disorders in the years 1867–71 is recorded. This shows an increasing percentage of those treated to be attributable to hemp. He also takes the trouble to reproduce 'a reference to the Annual Report of the Lunatic Asylums in Bengal for 1871 – Dullunda, Dacca, Patna, Moydapore', and finds that 'cannabis constitutes 31 per cent of the whole; 78 of the known causes of insanity.'[57]

Indeed the Resolution by the Government of India itself on the inquiry which was finally decided upon in December of 1873 reproduced the asylum statistics provided to it by the regional administrations. All of the above examples are mentioned in the resolution, including a reproduction of the table of Dr Penny and the direct quotes mentioned earlier.[58] The conclusion of the resolution, drawing on the statistical evidence reproduced from the asylum reports, states confidently of hemp that 'there can, however, be no doubt that its habitual use does tend to produce insanity ... of the cases of insanity produced by the excessive use of drugs or spirits, by far the largest number must be attributed to the abuse of hemp.'[59]

The Indian Hemp Drugs Commission (IHDC)

As mentioned this 1871/2 report which was very much the product of the categorization and enumeration process described was lodged in the House of Commons library by William Caine MP in 1893. It was Caine who asked the question in April of that year which lead to the House of Commons establishing the Indian Hemp Drugs Commission. The irony of the IHDC was that the process which lead to the establishment of the Commission was identified and heavily criticized within the final report of the Commission.

The report first recognized the importance of mental health institutions in the process of generating the issue of cannabis use and cannabis users as a concern for British government:

> Every asylum in British India was visited either by the Commission or by some members of the Commission and careful enquiries were conducted on the spot in every case of insanity attributed to the use of hemp drugs for a given period. The period selected was the calendar year 1892, the last for which statistics were available at the commencement of the Commission's labours.[60]

The report then identified the source of the information supplied to the medical officers at the asylums as to the cause of the state of mind of the new admission:

> The inquiry into the history of the case is not an inquiry conducted by a professional man from the persons likely to know most about the lunatic. The information consists often merely of the guesses of police officers as to the history and the habits of a friendless and homeless wanderer; and in other cases, where a local inquiry is possible, it is generally made by a subordinate police officer ... It would be absurd to accept without great distrust the statements, especially as to the cause of insanity, compiled by such an agency as has been described.[61]

Those on the Commission also identified the forces acting on the police officers to make sure that the forms were correctly completed. They cited the example provided by a Commissioner of Excise in Assam[62] who recounted stories of instructions being issued to impose fines on subordinate police officers for failing to supply the necessary information. He also pointed to the action taken by Indian officials at the asylums who felt compelled to provide information where none was forthcoming, 'a striking illustration of the effect of this pressure is found in the Dullunda Asylum returns for the following year (1863) in which the cause in several cases dating from the year 1857 and onwards was later changed from "unknown" to "ganja-smoking".'[63]

If the Commission discovered that the information being supplied to medical officers was coming from non medical officers they also discovered that these medical officers were happy to believe this information. Surgeon-Major Willcocks at Agra provided the following testimony:

> Ordinarily it has been the practice to enter hemp drugs as the cause of insanity where it has been shown that the patient used these drugs. I cannot say precisely why this is the practice. It has come down as the traditional practice. As a matter of fact until recently I looked upon these drugs as very poisonous. As I have already said, my ordinary medical practice did not bring me into contact with them at all. I only came into contact with them in the asylum. I had no idea that they were used as extensively as I find on enquiry to be the case.[64]

Dr Crombie of the Dacca asylum had published an article in the *Indian Medical Gazette* in 1892 which explained the statistical evidence of the asylums and showed how this proved that hemp drugs caused insanity. However he was forced by the Commission to agree that his conclusions were unreliable and admitted that his observations were almost entirely based on encounters in the asylum, 'in my practice outside of lunatic asylums my experience is confined to very few cases, only two or three in the whole course of my service, of ganja intoxication brought to hospital.'[65] In other words the process already identified in this article was picked out by the IHDC, where medical officers came to base their opinions of hemp preparations and hemp users in general entirely upon the information and experience of the asylums which was demonstrably inaccurate and unrepresentative.

If the Commission identified parts of the process whereby hemp users became categorized as a social menace in the imagination of the colonial medical officers it also pointed to the importance of the asylum statistics in translating localised suspicion into a governmental concern:

> There has been undoubtedly a popular impression that hemp drugs do cause insanity... besides this popular impression there has been great prominence given to asylum statistics as affording some tangible ground for judging of the effects of hemp drugs. Over and over again the statistics of Indian asylums have been referred to in official documents or scientific treatises not only in this country but also in other countries where the use of drugs has demanded attention.[66]

Indeed the Commission reiterated its belief in the influence of the numbers generated by the asylums in going as far as to say that 'hitherto any opinion regarding the connection between hemp drugs and insanity which has professed to have any solid basis at all or to be more than a vague impression has been based on the figures contained in the annual Statement no. VII appended to the Asylum reports.'[67]

The Commission then went on to object to these statistics which it considered to be difficult to consider trustworthy.[68] The first reason that it rubbished the numbers was that mentioned above, that the source of the information from which the statistics were compiled was questionable. Secondly, they found that administrative interference or errors also tended to inflate the number of cannabis related cases. The report included a case to show where there were discrepancies between what was on the descriptive roll which accompanied the admission from the police or the magistrate and what was included on the asylum register: 'Dr Macnamara, Superintendent of the Tezpur Asylum says: "the cause is entered in the general register from the police statement i.e. from the descriptive roll. We have nothing whatever to do with it. It is entered by the Overseer in charge of the Asylum, and ought to correspond with the entry of the descriptive roll". As a matter of fact, eleven of the thirteen cases for 1892 showed entries regarding cause which did not correspond with the descriptive rolls; and of these 11, no less than 10 were made, not by the Overseer but by his subordinate, the jemedar.'[69] Similarly they reproduced a case of apparent carelessness:

> Moung Min Thay was admitted on 25th June 1871. There has been no improvement in his mental state. There are no papers in his case except an order from the Magistrate to receive the man 'supposed to be insane'. The original entry in the case book shows cause as 'predisposing disease of the brain, exciting drinks, and smokes opium', and it shows the duration as 'probably from birth'. It also shows that the man was epileptic. There is no mention of ganja. The register for 1885 (the first to show causation) shows 'alleged duration' as 'congenital' and 'alleged cause' as 'drink and opium smoking'. The entry 'congenital' is continued until 1892 when it is replaced by a 'Do' under the 'Not Given' of a previous case. In 1886 the 'cause' similarly undergoes undesigned alteration. The word 'drink' is replaced by 'ganja' and in 1888 the reference to 'opium' is finally dropped. The case thus became a ganja case, and has been shown as such ever since. These all may be instances of exceptional carelessness but as a general rule it cannot be said that these entries have been made with care. Superintendents have not attached much importance to them. It has been left to subordinates to do this work; and that work as a rule has not been carefully supervised.[70]

Indeed when the Commission went back through the records of those in the asylums apparently admitted in 1892 due to behaviour caused by hemp preparations they found that of the 222 cases across India attributed to use of cannabis only 98 could be regarded as in any way reliable. The Commission had acknowledged that the asylum statistics were an important factor in establishing a connection between hemp use, hemp users, violence and madness. However they were far from convinced that these statistics could be relied upon.

In other words the final report of the IHDC concerned itself with exposing the process of categorization and enumeration which had lead to the establishment of the IHDC. It therefore concluded that 'there was no trustworthy basis for a satisfactory and reasonably accurate opinion on the connection between hemp drugs and insanity in the asylum statistics appended to the annual reports.'[71] It also pointed out that, 'as a rule these drugs do not tend to crime and violence.'[72] The prejudices of its members however meant that despite the lack of evidence to support the theory and despite the attempts at qualification[73] the IHDC still concluded that 'admitting (as we must admit) that hemp drugs as intoxicants cause more or less cerebral stimulation, it may be accepted as reasonably proved in the absence of other cause that hemp drugs do cause insanity.'

In other words the IHDC had demonstrated that the evidence built up since at least the 1870s to support the theory that hemp use was a sure route to insanity was based upon bad information, poor administration and the nature of colonial governmental systems. Yet its members could not escape their assumptions about the inevitability of harmful effects from freely available stimulants, assumptions that had been slowly embedding themselves in the belief systems of the British middle classes since the gin scares of the eighteenth century.[74]

Conclusion

Indians used hemp narcotics for a variety of reasons and it is entirely possible that its use at certain times disagreed with certain individuals to the extent that they became muddled or even murderous. Yet the few of those that did become muddled or murderous and that were snared in the net of the colonial state came to be taken as representative of all those in India that used cannabis preparations. From this, colonial government developed an image of all Indian users of hemp narcotics as dangerous, lunatic and potentially violent.

The reason that this image developed in the imagination of so many in the British administration was that the fantasies of those filling in the documents at the asylums were not dismissed as such. The reason for this was that the asylum, like the prisons explored by David Arnold, was one of the few sites available to the British for observing members of Indian society. Such observations were of course considered vitally important at a time when modern government was coming to rely on information about the governed as a tool of effective administration.[75] This chapter then has shown how the conclusions reached by individual officials in the isolated medical institutions of a colonial government, conclusions which were the result of administrative expedience, prejudices about intoxicants, mistrust of Indians and so on, could become issues which exercised colonial government and even metropolitain politicians. The asylum turns out to be a point of contact between Indian society and a colonial government geared to gathering knowledge from such points in order to make its rule more efficient and armed with the meta-language of statistics to translate the particular and the local observations into readily understandable and communicable generalizations.

The chapter however has done rather more than establish that. The issue of cannabis users and cannabis use as a social problem entrenched itself to the extent that those in colonial government had to be seen to act. Those in government in India developed colony wide policies aimed at restricting the use of the drug with a ban imposed in Burma and punitive levies introduced on sales of the drug in India. At the local level officials concerned themselves with controlling its users, 'many a man, reeling about the bazaar intoxicated with ganjah or spirit, finds himself, in coming to his senses, an inmate of a lunatic asylum.'[76] This local process of policing and surveillance explains case notes at the Lucknow asylum such as the following:

> Easeen Khan. Dementia. mussl. labourer. 32. 1 October 1861
> 1861 Oct. Sent in by City Magistrate, had been addicted to the use of ganja + on admission was suffering from its effects. As soon as these wore off, he appeared to be perfectly sane + on the 18th October was discharged.[77]

The simple fact that he was known to be a regular user of hemp narcotics is the only reason given for his incarceration. Indeed there is not even evidence of violent actions to call him to the attention of the authorities (the dementia diagnosis suggests that he had rendered himself insensible through the use of the drug).

In other words this chapter has not simply traced the development of a harmless misunderstanding or a bewildering self deception on the part of the British. It has examined the origins of a set of understandings of Indian society which lead to certain Indian practices and habits becoming demonised by the British authorities and to certain Indian individuals being harassed and incarcerated. The British had the power to look at and to judge Indians at the asylums and the last two chapters have outlined some of the images and the fantasies which were the result of this. But British power extended beyond simply generating this knowledge. The colonizers reimposed these images on India by actually seeking to reorder the societies that they imagined Indians to live in and by going out of their institutional observatories to arrest and harass real people who the British mistook for the fantasy figures that they had devised. The knowledge that they created at the asylum may have been no reflection of reality. But the British in their policies and their arrests certainly acted towards the population as if it was. This issue of the British power to interfere with and impose on India will be considered at the asylum in the next four chapters.

3
Disciplining Populations: British Admissions to 'Native-Only' Lunatic Asylums

Routes into the asylum

There were various routes by which an Indian could be admitted to a lunatic asylum in the period 1859–80. The *Rules for the Management and Control of the Lunatic Asylum at Lucknow*, included in the published responses to Sir James Clark's enquiry[1] into the treatment of lunatics in India, give a fair summary of these routes:

> The authorities empowered to order the admission of lunatics are:
> *First* – Officers exercising the powers of a Magistrate, in respect of wandering or dangerous lunatics, or lunatics who are neglected or maltreated (Sections 4+5 of Act XXXVI of 1858).
> *Second* – Judges of the principal Civil Courts of Districts, in respect of all other lunatics except the two classes hereafter mentioned (Section 8 of Act XXXVI of 1858).
> *Third* – The Local Government as regards criminal lunatics (Sections 390, 394, 396 of the Criminal Procedure Code).
> *Fourth* – Military Officers commanding Divisions, in respect of native non-commissioned officers and soldiers afflicted with insanity (Section 41, page 291 Bengal Military Regulations).
> *Fifth* – The Inspector of Jails, as regards the removal of any lunatic from one public asylum to any other within the circle of his inspection (Section 11, Act XXXVI of 1858).

Elsewhere in the Rules there are further details provided about criminal lunatics:

> Persons confined under the provisions of Chapter XXVII of the Criminal Procedure Code, whether unsentenced but found guilty of the act charged (Section 394) or already sentenced (Section 396) or found unsound of mind on trial by the Court of Sessions (Section 389) or deemed of unsound

mind by the Magistrate after recording the examination of the Civil Surgeon of the district or some other Medical Officer (Section 388) shall be admitted into the asylum under the order of the Local Government to which the case shall be reported through the usual channel by the Magistrate or Court of Sessions, or other officer, as the case may be (Section 390+394).[2]

The distinction between the criminal lunatic and the lunatic admitted as neglected, dangerous or wandering is one that was central in asylum administration. The Lucknow rules state that 'All criminal lunatics will be provided with a distinguishing dress, and will be confined apart from other lunatics in the enclosure and cells provided for them. Criminal male lunatics sentenced to rigorous imprisonment will wear a light iron ring on the left leg, and will be locked up at night.' Dr Corbyn at the Bareilly asylum mentioned that 'Criminal Lunatics are of course kept apart from the others, and have a yard and ward exclusively their own.'[3] It is not always clear that distinguishing dress, leg irons and spatial separation were enforced in other asylums. However it is certainly the case that by the 1860s the criminal lunatic as a separate subgroup of the asylum population was recognized throughout the asylums of British India. This is shown in the annually published reports supplied by the superintendents of each asylum in which a count of the criminal lunatics was routinely provided for each asylum, often with further statistics regarding their crimes, their marital status and so on. This division, between the criminal and the non-criminal, will initially be followed here.

It is apparent from the routes detailed above that the population within the asylums in British India was the product of the operation of a range of governmental organizations. This chapter will explore why the police, the medical, the penal and judicial agencies in the Government of India all produced candidates from within the Indian population for incarceration in the lunatic asylums.

The non-criminal lunatics

Act XXXVI of 1858 governed the admission of non-criminal lunatics into the asylums of British India. It stated in Clause IV that

it shall be the duty of every Darogah or District Police Officer to apprehend and send to the Magistrate all persons found wandering at large within his district who are deemed to be Lunatics and all persons believed to be dangerous by reasons of Lunacy. Whenever any such person as aforesaid is brought before a Magistrate, the Magistrate, with the assistance of a Medical Officer, shall examine such person, and if the Medical Officer shall sign a certificate in the Form A in the schedule to this Act, and the Magistrate shall be satisfied on personal examination or other proof that such person is a Lunatic and a proper person to be detained under care and treatment, he shall make an order for such Lunatic to be received into the Asylum established for that Division.

and established in Clause V that

if it shall appear to the Magistrate, on the report of a Police Officer or the information of any other person, that any person within the limits of his jurisdiction deemed to be a Lunatic is not under proper care and control, or is cruelly treated or neglected by any relative or other person having the charge of him, the Magistrate may send for the supposed Lunatic and summon such relative or other person as has or ought to have the charge of him . . . If there be no person legally bound to maintain the supposed Lunatic, or if the Magistrate thinks fit so to do, he may proceed as prescribed in the last preceding Section.[4]

Wanderers, the dangerous and the neglected were the targets of this legislation although there is evidence that the authorities charged with putting the legislation into practice subsequently refined this. For example, it is doubtful if the Police regularly concerned themselves with the treatment of the insane in Indian homes, as Dr Simpson of the Dacca asylum wrote in 1862: 'With Native Police this section becomes null and void.'[5] There is no evidence in the whole of the Lucknow case notes of a patient having been admitted as a result of poor treatment by his/her family becoming the concern of the authorities, and indeed there are case notes such as the following which suggest the opposite:

Allo Rukee (f). Dementia. 26. Mussl. Beggar. 7th February/65.
7th February 1865. Sent in by City Magistrate of Lucknow.
2nd April 1865. This appears to be a case of melancholy mania probably the effects of bad treatment at home. No improvement whatever.
29th August 1865. Made over to her husband much improved.[6]

That she was dismissed as 'much improved' rather than with the more common 'discharged, cured' would suggest that the medical officer writing the report still considered her less than completely free of the symptoms which had led to the original diagnosis but was looking for a satisfactory formulation to justify releasing a harmless but disordered and demoralized woman. Significantly though, he released her back to the very family which it was reckoned had treated her so poorly. In other words this would appear to be an example of a process which was the exact reverse of that which it was deemed desirable in law to follow: a lunatic was being released back into a family which it was felt neglected her.

Indeed, notes of concern in official correspondence in the 1860s suggest that this was not just the case in Lucknow and that elsewhere the authorities were failing to implement the part of the act relating to maltreated lunatics in Indian homes. For example, some ten years after the Act the opinion of the superintendent of Moydapore in Bengal was being reproduced in official correspondence:

> It is I think, allowed by all who have any intimate knowledge of the village population of this country that the number of lunatics in our asylums represents a very small proportion of that unfortunate class to be found in every district; and that the vastly larger proportion is kept at home and supposed to be taken care of by their relatives; but this care consists of a degree of severity towards them, especially if they have the least tendency to be obstreperous.[7]

The filtering into asylums of those insanes neglected in their homes envisaged by the 1858 Act seems largely to have been forgotten or sidelined in the actual admission of non-criminal lunatics. By far the largest proportion of this group was made up by what can be termed public order problems: the wanderers and the dangerous.

The wanderers

> Ram Deen. Mania. 35. Hindoo. Kapoor. 12th Feby/63.
> Sent in by Cantonment Magistrate – was found wandering about Suddur Bazar at night. He talks + mutters very great nonsense, is apparently harmless.
> 1864. This man was never in the enjoyment of good health. Always looked sickly + did not improve in his mental condition about 6 weeks ago he began to suffer from Diarrhoea – it gradually reduced him + became intractable. Died on 14th July 1864.[8]

The example of Ram Deen closely followed the example of Gosalee in the case book for 1863:

> Gosalee. Maniah. 28. Hindoo. Beggar. 8th Jan'63.
> Sent in by City Mag. of Lucknow found knocking about the city calls himself 'Moonshie Ram Dyal.' Is very wild and displays much excitement and general incoherence in making replies to questions.
> June 1863. Died of chronic diarrhoea.[9]

Indeed of the first seven admissions of 1863 of which these two are examples, five were admitted in similar circumstances. These circumstances suggested little about their mental state. That the British superintendent who filled in the case notes could make no sense of Ram Deen's mumblings or Gosalee's anger is hardly evidence of insanity. Both sets of behaviour might be understood less as symptoms of madness and more as the result of the fear and indignation at being summarily arrested by the authorities of poor Indians used to minding their own business.

Instead of revealing much about their mental state, the circumstances of their detention seem to point to the social status of Ram Deen and Gosalee. These admissions were vagrants. Indeed it does not appear to be the case that 1863 was a particularly bad year to be a wanderer in India. Throughout the case notes for the period 1860 to 1872 similar examples crop up. A year before in 1862 there is the case of Allee Jaim:

> Allee Jaim. Mania. Mussl. Beggar. 40. 19 Feby 1862.
> Feb 1812. This man was sent in by City Magistrate of Lucknow – he had been taken up by Police as a beggar – whether from want or dissipation he appears to be weak in intellect and is so reduced in flesh + natural vigour that it is evident he has not long to live. Suffered from diarrhoea ever since admission – gradually got weaker + died 25th March 1862.[10]

Indeed, entries still read like this in the following decade:

> Mosst.Khunnia. Chronic Mania. 23. Hindoo. Labour. 29th April 1870. Certified by the magistrate 'not violent.'
> 1870 April 29. Sent in from Roy Bareilly – has been wandering about that district for years picking up her living how she could, she appears a harmless, quiet individual.[11]

What these case notes have in common is the scarcity of information about their mental states. As already stated, the little evidence of behaviour that is produced to demonstrate the 'insanity' of the admitted individuals is more readily understandable as the fear or anger of someone suddenly arrested. Indeed in the final example there is no reference whatsoever by the medical officer to the mental state of the inmate. From what details there are on the case note she simply appears to be a woman who had always kept herself to herself on the margins of the society in the area that she lived.

The first conclusion then to be drawn from these case notes is that there is little evidence of the insanity of those being incarcerated where vagrancy is suggested on the document. These people hardly seem 'mad' from these documents, just frightened or upset individuals caught up in the machinery of the state. The second conclusion, and perhaps the more important one, is that there was little time or interest devoted by the authorities to establishing that these people were insane. It is by no means clear then that 'madness' was the reason for the incarceration of these individuals or indeed that it was considered necessary to convincingly demonstrate that it was the reason for incarceration.

A look at the case notes of further detainees where there is evidence that links their lifestyle to vagrancy suggests the reason that so little attention was paid to mental state on such case notes. Banda ally Khan was classified as a beggar on his document which opened with the following details: 'This man was sent in by the City Magistrate. He had been found in the streets and could give no satisfactory account of himself. On admission he appeared to be labouring under the effects of some intoxicating drug.'[12] Among these details, which basically seem to record an inebriated vagrant rather than a 'madman' is the key phrase that Banda ally Khan 'could give no satisfactory account of himself.' This is a phrase encountered in other case notes. Boodhoo for example was 'found in the bazaar and unable to give any account of himself'[13] and Jookea, a female admission 'sent in by City Magistrate of Lucknow was found wandering about the streets, could give no account of herself, is young and good-looking.'

The significance of this phrase of course was that it appeared in Section 295 of the Code of Criminal Procedure (CPC) of 1861:

> Whenever it shall appear to the Magistrate of the District or to an officer exercising the powers of a Magistrate that any person is lurking within his jurisdiction not having any ostensible means of subsistence, or who cannot give a satisfactory account of himself, it shall be competent to such Magistrate or other officers as aforesaid to require security for the good behaviour of such person for a period not exceeding six months.[14]

The penalty for failing to provide security for good behaviour could be imprisonment. This was legislation designed to give the authorities the power to control vagrancy and it is significant that the same language appears on case notes at a lunatic asylum to justify the detainment of certain individuals. The implication is that the medical officer had in mind Section 295 when making the decision to incarcerate these individuals. Vagrancy rather than insanity was his concern when writing the case notes for wandering individuals.

Section 295 of the CPC alongside the provisions for detaining vagrants in Act XXXVI of 1858, mentioned above, gave the colonial authorities the power to detain all those individuals that they considered to be 'wandering' or 'lurking' in their districts. These legislative provisions dealing with individuals should be seen alongside legislation like the Criminal Tribes Act of 1871 which originally applied just in the North-Western Provinces, the Punjab and Oudh.[15] This act was aimed at providing the legal framework within which the colonial state could prevent the movement of whole groups of Indians. The nomadic lifestyles of the communities identified in these acts were rendered illegal by the colonial state and systems were established to manage and prevent those lifestyles. Provisions included having suspect tribes register themselves in fixed places and necessitated the possession of a license before travelling.

This preoccupation with dealing with vagrants seemed so pressing sometimes to officials on the ground that it often lead them to go beyond the measures set up by legislative means or by government policy. Examples like those in Oudh show how illegal arrest and detention was used as a solution to the mobility of certain Indian communities. The Chief Commissioner noted in 1880 that he had

> received a petition from some Barwars complaining of the persecution they are subjected to, and asserting that two hundred of their castemen, being a very large proportion of the males of the tribe, are undergoing imprisonment without having been convicted of any special offence under the Penal Code.[16]

He explained that it was believed by the British that this group, 'by tradition worship a deity of theft' and 'that they are of roving habits.'[17] However, these people were not members of a British classified wandering tribe but they had become linked in the British imagination with a deity of theft. Therefore even if they appeared 'industrious and have business at fairs and such places'[18] they were regarded with suspicion. This explains why Barwars while travelling for whatever reason were simply picked up and incarcerated by colonial officials who had no legal grounds for detaining them. This system of illegal detention, the Chief Commissioner admitted was little more than 'a mode of indiscriminate terrorism'[19] on the part of the district authorities.

While local officials were able to improvise strategies for dealing with itinerant communities it appears that they were sufficiently concerned with individual vagrants to make sure that they did not slip through the net either. Examples like that of Angnoo are interesting in this context. Although ultimately a patient in the asylum, it appears that the original arrest was not made with the asylum in mind. In other words it is not at all clear that he was arrested because obviously insane and therefore a candidate for treatment in the specialist institution. Rather the details read as if he was detained because he was found 'in the district' and was then shuffled through the system until somewhere to detain him was found:

> Angnoo. Dementia. Hindoo. Barber. 25. 14 October 1861.
> 1861. Sent in by police. His papers were irregular and returned to City Magistrate for correction, but they were never received.
> He had been picked up in the district + forwarded from thannah to thannah until brought to the asylum. He was in very low state of health, scarcely ate any food + could with difficulty be managed. He had diarrhoea or fever which improved by good food. During the cold weather however, it returned + became quite intractable. Died 26th March 1862.[20]

Similarly the example of Punchum shows how the detention of an individual resulted in that individual being shunted between institutions and agencies. Although a range of specialist facilities was available, the jail of the police, the city hospital and the asylum in this case, the detainee was not arrested and then accepted at any one of these. In other words it does not look like the arrest was made with a specific problem, crime, illness or insanity in mind. Rather the arrest was simply made to halt the mobility of the individual and the process then began of trying to find a space in the network of institutions where that detainee might be stowed away:

> Punchum. Mania. Hindoo. Faqueer. 60. 27th Novr.
> 1861 Nov. This man was admitted from City Hospital. He was brought there by the Police and no history of his case was procurable. Was in a very weakly state. Was quite unable to take food + died 2nd Dec. 1860.[21]

It seems then that the authorities were keen to stop individual Indians from wandering about and having arrested them to prevent them from doing so the authorities found themselves having to improvise an institutional solution to the problem of where to put those they considered vagrants having taken them off the street. Indeed this determination to improvise an institutional response to the perceived problem of individual wanderers is sometimes evident on a larger scale. Because it was pointed out that 'the district authorities naturally find it difficult to take care of harmless idiots found wandering about without any means of subsistence and whose relatives cannot be found', the Chief Commissioner of Oudh went ahead and

> sanctioned the construction of three barracks in the enclosure of the Lunatic Asylum to provide for the accommodation of twenty-four male and twelve female idiots. These buildings will be constructed from provincial funds, but the charge for the care and maintenance of each idiot will be borne by the local funds of the district from which the idiot was sent to the asylum.[22]

This local decision to provide another institution at the government's expense to contain a group of individual vagrants flew in the face of 'instructions of the Government of India interdicting the practice of sending incurable and harmless idiots to the Lunatic Asylum.'[23] These instructions had been issued on the grounds that it 'does not seem desirable in any way to increase unnecessarily the charges upon the State for Lunatic Asylums' and it appears from the correspondence in Oudh about the subject that the authorites there were perfectly aware of the Government of India's policy.[24] In other words, the local government in Oudh was so preoccupied with the problem of detaining individual vagrants that they went as far as to found an institution in open defiance of the orders of the superior authority of the Government of India.

Overall then a picture emerges of a network of colonial officers, from those in the towns and the districts to those in the Government of India and the legislative council, which concerned itself with the mobility of the Indian population. This concern expressed itself in the range of strategies devised to control that mobility, from the legislative acts of the GOI to the local and sometimes illegal arrests made by the local magistrates. This concern can be explained in two ways. The first explanation is that government in Britain had occupied itself even in pre-modern times with the problem of mobile populations which were difficult to tax and to keep under surveillance.[25] With the advent of the industrial age this suspicion in government of itinerant lifestyles intensified. Vagrancy was routinely associated with wilful poverty at a time when the authorities imagined that 'pauperism was a rejection of regular employment which meant also an existence outside the benign self-regulating mechanisms of the economy . . . a refusal of all those relations which were so essential to a healthy, wealthy and well-ordered polity.'[26]

Yet a long history of concern with mobile groups and individuals in systems of British government only partly explains the importance placed on restricting such people by the colonial authorities in India. In 1857/8 the British had lost control of much of rural north India to roaming bands of peasants and mutinous soldiers and had been besieged in the cities by the local population. This had demonstrated to the colonial authorities the limits of their ability to monitor and check threats to their rule and had emphasized their isolation and vulnerability as a small group in India's large population. After 1857 then a range of policies were adopted to render Indian movement more transparent to surveillance and easier to organize. These policies ranged from those already mentioned, which were aimed at controlling the movement of specific groups and individuals around the towns and the countryside, to the complete spatial reorganization of cities. This meant demolishing the winding streets and tight bazaars of Indian cities and replacing them with wide boulevards and orderly shopping streets. The effect of this was to make Indian movement more visible and easier to anticipate.[27]

There are certainly suggestions in the evidence above that individual officers may have resisted having their institution cluttered up with people who they regarded as having no place in a hospital or asylum or lock-up or whichever. This would explain why certain patients were moved on from 'thannah to thannah', from hospital to asylum and indeed why even at the asylum there was felt the need for a separate 'idiot-ward' in which those wanderers deemed unfit for asylum living might be detained. Not all officers were keen to use all the resources available to them to control the vagrancy problem.

The overall picture however is of an institutional network in which individual vagrants were being incarcerated as part of a wider determination on the part of many British officers in India after 1857 to limit the mobility of the Indian population. The asylum was part of that institutional network and many of the admissions were victims of that British determination. This explains why many examples of case notes from Lucknow contain little if any information on the possibility of detainees being 'insane' but so often refer to the wandering circumstances of the individual when picked up. It seems then that those writing up the case notes of these inmates were more preoccupied with the vagrancy of the new admission than with his/her state of mind.

The Dangerous

It is not easy to discover the details of behaviour in most of the cases admitted as 'violent' or 'dangerous' as they usually read like that of Nuncoo:

> Nuncoo. Dementia. 26. Hindoo. Cultivator. 25 June/64.
> 25 June 1864. Sent in by Deputy Commr. of Baraitch.
> 25 March 1865. She remains a violent lunatic + is in no respect improved.
> 26th August 1866. Died of chronic diarrhoea.[28]

With so little information about such admissions it is difficult to ascertain what type of behaviour lead to the original incarceration. If wildly disruptive and aggressive, the only information available about her is that the medical officer writing the case note thought that she continued to be so. One case note does exist which contains rather more detail about the behaviour of an inmate incarcerated as he was considered dangerous. This is the case note of Jeobodh Koomar, an inmate of the Lucknow asylum for almost thirty years:

> ~~Amentia~~. Mania ~~acute~~ chronic. Jeobodh Koomar. 28. Hindoo. Daily Labourer. 27th Feb. 1869. Certified by Magistrate Violent.
> 27th Feb/69. Sent in by the Magistrate of Fyzabad, there is no previous history of this man's health and habits – he appears to me to be a very excitable idiot, that may prove violent and even dangerous at times – his habits are very filthy. The Civil Surgeon of Fyzabad certified 22 Feb. 1869, 'Jeobodh sits in his cell occasionally beating himself against the wall. Dirty in habits. Smears himself over with his faeces, general aspect that of a maniac. Said to attempt to bite all who approach him. Will not always speak + when does, gives incoherent answers. Does not eat unless fed.'
> 1st June 1872. A congenital idiot – no improvement.
> 10th Feby 1873. Just the same as last report.
> Oct 11. This man has attained excellence in durrie weaving. He is very industrious.
> 1878 Aug 1st. He has a scar on his forehead. When asked how he got mark he said, 'When I was working in field.' He is now in a great rage, and utters every kind of abuse in a furious manner. 'Everybody knows my name Jeobodh as a man who can do everything. God made me stand upright.' He refers in a loud, screaming voice + extreme anger to my having put him into a bag for violence. When I smiled he said as much as, 'Go on laugh, I will make you cry.'
> They say he is never violent except when he sees Europeans though sometimes he gets angry. He has not been so angry for a very long time. They say he sometimes gets abortive attacks of epilepsy. The Hosp.Asst. has not seen them.
> 1884 March 29. Continues to get excited. Works well – General health good.
> 1888 June 11. Is in poor health.
> 17 June. Is satisfied to remain where he is. He works regularly and there is no change in his condition.

1889 14 April. Is very quiet and has lately been attending to the cows. He is thin and suffers dysentery. Ordered 2 chittacks meat and 1/2 oz.ghee.

5 Aug. Is now in good condition. Extra food is stopped. Is mentally the same.

1893 15 Jan. So often excited and noisy. Gets milk. In fair condition. Weighs 108 lbs.

May 1895. Suffers from periodic attacks of mania which last for about a week. In the intervals he works in the weaving factory. General health fair. Weight 102, 6lbs. less than when last weighed. Is given a little more extra food.

May 1895. This man has been losing weight; now 94lbs. Gets extra diet. Mental condition the same.

March 1896. Old and decrepit – has been in hospital for neuralgia of stomach since 19 Jan. 1896.[29]

It is worth quoting the entire length of this case as it provides clues as to the nature of the behaviour likely to lead to detainment as a 'dangerous' lunatic. The broad impression from the case note is that this man was subject to occasional temporary rages. He first came to the attention of the authorities when he was brought to the Civil Surgeon of Fyzabad during one of his attacks. However, he seems to have calmed down sufficiently by the time that the superintendent of the asylum wrote his first report for the author to decide that he was only 'dangerous at times' and that he was no more than an excitable simpleton.

The issue here though is what happens between 1873 and 1878, between 1878 and 1884 and in the period 1884 to 1888. These lengthy silences on the case note suggest that Jeeobodh Kumar did nothing to bring himself to the attention of the superintendent who has had nothing to note on the document. Indeed in these lengthy periods of time he seemed able to learn new skills and to work in an orderly and productive manner. Despite these long periods of calm and despite his apparent ability to fend for himself he was never released.

The only explanation for his being kept in the asylum for almost thirty years despite these lengthy periods of calm is that the superintendent was wary of his *potential* for violence. He was not incarcerated because he was permanently furious or aggressive. He was detained and remained an inmate as the authorities feared the latent danger he represented, especially as it was feared that his unpredictable violence would be aimed at Europeans.

The incarceration of those who were not permanently aggressive but who had demonstrated the potential for violence is evident in other case notes:

Bholai. Chronic Mania. 40. Ahir. Cult. 9th Feby. 1869. Certified magistrate – violent/dangerous, throws bricks at people.
9th Feby 1869. Bholai admitted for first time. Is said to be occasionally very violent and filthy. To be kept with the violent lunatics – sent
in by Magistrate of Sultanpoor.[30]

And also in inmates admitted throughout the period:

Subnee. Mania. Hindoo. Beggar. 25. 21 October.
1861. Sent by Police from Murnarra. Was very wild and excited, is
subject to occasional attacks of greater severity. Generally quiet and well-
behaved – spins – appears to have no friends and no enquiries have
ever been made after her.
1866. Died of debility on 1st September 1866.[31]

The significance of this example is again that there is a considerable silence between entries. The original pointed out that that the
inmate was 'wild and excited' and the subsequent note which came
five years later recorded her death. In other words for the best part
of half a decade she seems to have done nothing to bring herself
to the attention of the asylum management. It is true that at one
point she was sufficiently angry about something to be 'very wild
and excited.' All the evidence suggests however that this was a temporary rage and that once calm again she remained so. Her potential
to be violent however, this allegation that she was 'subject to occasional attacks of greater severity', seems to have sealed her fate
despite all the evidence that on the whole she was generally 'quiet
and well behaved.'

These patients all seem to be subject to occasional, intense and
temporary paroxysms of intense and aggressive behaviour. It appears then that the British used their asylums less to incarcerate
those who were a permanent danger by way of their constant ag-
gression and more to detain those who although usually 'quiet and
well-behaved' were seen as a future threat to public order as they
had demonstrated a potential for sudden, very physical, fury.

Removing such people from Indian society can be seen in the
context of policies aimed at rendering the Indian population do-
cile. Such policies were part of the period when 'the Indian people
were being systematically disarmed.'[32] This description is usually
taken to refer to the disarming operations undertaken under the
Arms Acts XXVIII of 1857 and XXXI of 1860. The more extreme
measures of the first act legitimized searching out and confiscating
weapons, and even the second, less stringent act, authorized the

disarming of all whom the Magistrate considered 'a danger to the public peace.'[33]

These measures were the result of the anxieties of colonial rulers facing a largely unknown population. Knowing little about the Indian people meant that British had failed to anticipate the attacks on their rule of 1857. The colonizers therefore came to imagine the population to have a capacity for sudden and unpredictable violence. As such, the British were eager to take whatever steps they could to limit the threats that the Indian population could present. This meant doing anything from taking weapons away from Indians to actually removing potentially dangerous and unpredictable individuals from society. The broad objective of all such measures was to limit the violent surprises that the indigenous communities could throw at British rule. Thus those who came to the attention of the authorities as they had proven themselves even occasionally aggressive or disordered were detained in asylums as the British attempted to anticipate the dangers which they feared they faced.

The British attempted the legitimation of their non-criminal lunatic admission policies by claiming humanitarian motives. 'It is refreshing to think that the condition of insanes of this country attracts so much attention; for there is no doubt that their condition was very miserable, and that they were much neglected',[34] opined J. Penny, the superintendent of the asylum at Delhi. Beneath the humanitarian myth lay a series of strategies directed to disciplining, that is drilling and controlling, the colonized population as a whole. The incarceration of the non-criminal Indian lunatics was one of the many strategies devised by the authorities during this period to control the Indian population and to limit its potential for disorder. To a certain extent, what lay behind this range of disciplinary processes, from the incarceration of vagrants to the licensing of tribal group movements, lay the meta-narratives of modern governmental anxieties familiar from Britain: 'The ideology sustaining the notion of "criminal tribes" was not wholly a product of the colonial environment. Even in Victorian Britain the government feared the so called 'dangerous classes', who were conceived of as threatening public order.'[35]

What has been established though is that there was a peculiarly colonial narrative surrounding strategies such as the incarceration of those deemed 'wandering' or 'dangerous.' This was the insecurity of the European community which, especially after 1857, determined the disarmament of the Indian population, the transformation of physical spaces to segregate Indians from Europeans[36] and indeed the reconfiguration of social and cultural spaces to enforce the distance of Indians from their colonizers.[37] Those admitted to the asylum were those whose lives seemed to represent to the British what they feared most in the Indian population; mobility and unfathomable unpredictability became 'wandering' and 'dangerous' on the case notes of the individuals in the asylum. It must be remembered though that the asylum was only one of a range of measures, some planned at government level like the Criminal Tribes Act, some improvised at the local level like an 'idiot ward' or a Poor House, which the colonizers devised to deal with such embodiments of their anxieties.

The criminal lunatics

A small but significant group of those admitted to the asylums has yet to be mentioned though. The number of criminal lunatics in the asylums is often difficult to calculate as the information available is patchy. However, it seems that by the end of the 1860s they made up almost a quarter of the population residing in the asylums in Bengal[38] and that by the end of the 1870s the criminal group constituted a third of the asylum population there.[39] This increase in significance of the group within the asylums is mirrored elsewhere, as figures available for the asylum in Oudh[40] show a steady increase from 1866 onwards of criminal class patients in the asylum and the two mental hospitals in the Central Provinces[41] show dramatic leaps in the proportion of patients admitted, treated and remaining who were criminal class. In other areas though it is a less straightforward task to identify a trend. The Bombay[42] figures for 1869 compared with 1879 suggest a drop in the percentage of those being admitted over the twelve month period who were criminal between the end of the 1860s and the end of the 1870s, and even when the totals for the last three years of each decade are averaged out it seems that at most the percentage has remained constant. The proportion of those remaining at the end of the year who were criminal shows only a slight increase from the last three years of the 1860s to those of the 1870s as well. This is similar to the situation in Madras.[43]

Perhaps the most significant set of figures though is those which show the proportion of the population incarcerated by the British in this period as criminals who were confined in the asylums as opposed to the lock-ups and prisons. Only in Bengal and the Central Provinces was more than 1 per cent of the total incarcerated criminal population resident in an asylum at the end of a year by the end of the 1870s. Figures available for the other provinces suggest in most cases a rise in the proportion of those confined being so in an asylum over the period (Bombay being a notable exception) but the figures remain extremely small.[44] Quite simply then only a tiny percentage of those that the British had incarcerated across India because they had been convicted of a crime ended up in asylums while the overwhelming majority of these passed their sentences in prison. The question remains then of what was so distinctive about those individuals which were singled out among those incarcerated for crime which made the authorities segregate them in a separate institution.

It has been suggested in studies made of the treatment of the criminal lunatic in England that, during this period, 'something of a stereotype of the criminal lunatic as a violent dangerous lunatic was elaborated' which was 'further enhanced by the legal fraternity's obsession with establishing links between insanity and violent crime.'[45] The popular market for psychiatric literary productions and the memoirs of ex-prisoners all helped to embellish this image of the violent criminal madman in the lay imagination. It could be then that this stereotype, firmly established in the culture of the British who acted as magistrates in India, was transported with them and took root in the criminal justice system that they operated. The British may simply have been locking away in the asylums of India the most violent and dangerous of the criminals that they came across in the belief that these people fitted the stereotype of the criminal madman.

When the crimes for which the criminals in asylums were being detained are listed this thesis could find support. It appears that passage into the asylum was helped if the crime was against the person. Figures on the crimes of those criminals in the asylum are only available in the records intermittently and the most complete figures are available for Bombay at the end of the 1870s. There crimes against the person (murder, grievous hurt, assaults, homicide, rape, suicide and so on) accounted for between two thirds and three quarters of those criminal lunatics treated in the four largest Bombay Presidency asylums in any one year. Murder is always the largest category of crime for which criminals are detained in the mental hospitals.

The problem with this explanation for criminal admissions to the Indian lunatic asylums is the very small number of those violent criminals actually to end up in an institution for insanes. It is difficult to track down the totals of those incarcerated in prisons at any one point for any one crime and have comparable statistics for the asylum. It is possible to note such figures though like that in the Bombay Presidency when there were 315 convictions for the violent crime of 'grievous hurt' in 1880 alone.[46] There was a grand total of only 18 criminals resident in asylums associated with this crime at the end of that year (note this is total resident not total admissions for the year, it is impossible to know how many of this number were admitted in 1880). There must be something distinctive about these 18 cases to distinguish them from the many others admitted to prison for the same crime but who never made it to the asylum. After all most incidents involving 'grievous hurt' are violent so the issue of whether these were simply the 18 most violent criminals or whether there were other factors which influenced the decision to admit these inmates to an asylum must be addressed.

Work done on the processes involving criminal lunatics in Victorian Britain emphasizes the importance of local factors and decisions which ultimately served to decide whether an individual found his/her way into an asylum. Using this focus in the Indian study it will be argued that the working of institutional management systems or of local administrative machinery is as important in explaining admissions to asylums in colonial south Asia as are over-arching meta-narratives of colonial anxiety or cultural conditioning.

Witnesses

The importance of witnesses at some stage in legal proceedings is focused on in British case studies. Nigel Walker includes in the two volume study *Crime and Insanity in England* the observation that 'until the 1860s when prison doctors were at last required to inspect every prisoner regularly the recognition of disorder depended largely on fortuitous circumstances.' One such set of circumstances was that, 'the prisoner might have relatives who could draw attention to his mental state.'[47] Joel Peter Eigen, in his recent study, stresses the importance of witness testimony in early nineteenth century trials where insanity was an issue and emphasizes the weight given to it in comparison to that given by so-called expert medical witnesses:

It is clear that neighbours, lovers and relatives of allegedly mad prisoners were appearing in court under much the same rubric as acquaintances of any prisoner whose past behaviour might be thought to have a bearing on the jury's deliberation – that is, as character witnesses. After all, acquaintances of sane prisoners appeared not as 'experts' in human character but as intimates of the accused, informing the court of the prisoner's habitual functioning.[48]

Despite the variety of this testimony, from a simple reference to neighbourhood knowledge to intimate accounts of life with the prisoner, it seems that the courts were prepared to take full account of such observations. Eigen concludes that 'whether it was a surfeit of folk wisdom that attended the experience of madness or a belief that it was not particularly mysterious but decipherable by the "inexperienced" eye, mad-doctors in court faced special obstacles. The observations of lay witnesses were apparently given the aura of officially sanctioned opinion.'[49]

Circumstances in India were certainly such that the presence of relatives or associates willing to point out that a prisoner had mental health problems could be decisive. Most doctors in charge of jails and lock ups would have had little or no expertise or training in the diagnosis of mental illness.[50] It was also the case that those given charge of a prison often had many other duties in a station. This would have meant that even those who did have specialist knowledge of mental illness would have been unlikely to have had sufficient time in contact with the inmates to notice those with symptoms.[51]

Added to these factors were the difficulties of cross-cultural diagnosis. The problems involved in determining 'insanity' in legal proceedings in the colonial environment have been discussed elsewhere and would certainly have featured in India in this period.[52] Although a person was acting in ways that were deemed so inappropriate within his/her own culture and community that he/she would have been seen as insane by that community there was no guarantee that a Western magistrate would know that this behaviour was judged as such. Only a representative of that community presenting him/herself as a witness to that insanity would have been able to alert the legal authorities to the possibility of madness complicating the case.

A series of examples from the records of the North-Western Provinces in the early 1860s are important here. They offer a glimpse of a system where the intervention of lay witnesses in the medico-legal process of establishing responsibility for a crime appears to have been the decisive element in determining the verdict.

For example, there is the case of Koonj Beharee Singh[53] who was accused of culpable homicide. On 25 March 1860 he was eating at the house of a local zamindar. The victim Dulgunjun, who was a Gorait, approached despite being forbidden by the defendant to do so. This disobedience resulted in the Gorait being clubbed on the head by the defendant. Dulgunjun's response to this assault was to announce his intention of reporting his assailant to the thannadar and to start out on this course. Koonj Beharee Singh thereupon chased the victim and dealt a fatal blow to the defendant with the same club.

In disposing of the case the Sessions Judge, one A. Swinton, decided that Koonj Beharee Singh's decision to attack the victim for a second time when faced with the prospect of being reported was a rational one. This was sufficient evidence of his sanity to hold him responsible for his action. He was sentenced to two years imprisonment and a fine of Rs 50.

However the Sudder Court acquitted him 'by reason of unsoundness of mind not wilfully caused by himself, he was unconscious and incapable of knowing at the time of committing the culpable homicide with which he is charged that he was doing an act forbidden by law.' The medical evidence for such a verdict is less than unequivocal. The Officiating Civil Surgeon deposed that

> I examined Koonj Beharee Singh on the 15th June and he was then in an unsound state of mind he had been under treatment for some weeks, during which time a considerable improvement had taken place. As there were very few signs of insanity, I think the aberration must have been of recent date. He did not show any violent symptoms, and gave incoherent replies to questions, and was occasionally restless, his acts betrayed symptoms of weakness of intellect. I do not consider he has completely recovered and it would be inadvisable at present to set him at liberty. I would recommend that he be forwarded to the Insane Hospital.

Elsewhere in the papers the Sessions Judge noted that 'Dowlut Ram, native doctor, deposed that defendant was insane when admitted into the hospital on 5th May 1860 and continued in that state 'til the end of August and did not recover his senses before the 1st September.' These testimonies do not assert that the defendant was insane *at the time* that the crime was committed. The only way to be aquitted of a crime on grounds of insanity was to prove that while the crime was being committed the defendant was insane.

The statements of lay witnesses though give every reason to suggest that he could have been insane at the time of the crime. Although only available in summary form, the flavour of the testimony is preserved. Goolzar Chumar, son of the victim, stated that the defendant seemed intoxicated. Another witness according to Swinton's summary deposed 'that defendant was seen smoking ganja at the time of the occurrence and was not in his proper senses.' Significantly, Mungra Koeree and Goopta Doobey 'depose to the fact of defendant being subject to fits of insanity for several years: they live in his village.'

While the medical staff involved state that on their seeing him (in both cases a number of weeks after the incident) he was insane, this falls far short of establishing that he was insane at the moment of the criminal act. What the lay witness testimony does is provide the grounds for backdating the official medical diagnosis to the time of the event. The suggestion that at the time of the crime he was smoking a drug widely believed by the British to be linked with insane behaviour[54] and that he was prone to insane episodes might have justified the extension of the medical officers' observations on his mental state back to the day of the crime. This in turn justified the acquittal on the grounds of insane at the time of the act.

An even clearer example of the central place of witness testimony in Indian criminal trials which feature insanity is the case of Kishore,[55] charged with the murder of his wife but acquitted on the ground of insanity. Consider the deposition of the medical officer involved in the case:[56]

Q. What is your name and profession?
A. William R. Rice, Civil Assistant Surgeon.
Q. Have you examined the prisoner Kishore, and if so, please state the result of your observations as to his state of mind?
A. When he first entered he appeared to be labouring under a little excitement which subsided in a day or two since that time he has shewn no signs of insanity. I consider his moral faculties to be inferior to the general order of men of the same class. That he is a man of excitable temper.
Q. Having heard the statements of the prisoners' relations as to his previous state of mind, and the insanity of his father, are you of opinion that he was labouring under a temporary fit of insanity at the time he committed this crime?
A. Yes. I am of opinion from the evidence I have heard given, that he was labouring under an irresistible impulse to destroy life in fact he was labouring under homicidal mania.

The impression which this exchange gives is of a medical officer who had noticed strange behaviour in a patient but who hesitated to call it insanity until the intervention of lay witnesses to positively identify the behaviour as such. Elsewhere in the papers R.B. Morgan, a judge, noted the following:

> The medical officer, although he pronounced him sane at the time his [Kishore's] deposition was recorded, stated that when he first examined the prisoner, he appeared to be labouring under a little excitement which subsided in a day or two, and having heard the statements of the prisoners' relations as to his previous state of mind, the Civil Surgeon was of opinion that the prisoner was labouring under an irresistible impulse to destroy life. It appears to me therefore that there is evidence sufficient on the record to enable us to pronounce that the prisoner was insane. That he was incapable of discriminating at the time that he was committing a criminal act.[57]

It was thought then that when Kishore gave his deposition the medical officer believed him sane. He only came to positively identify Kishore as insane as a result of the witness testimony. Moreover, for the legal authorities this testimony was perfectly ample by way of proof that the accused was insane at the moment of the act.

The witness testimony is only available in the summary of the Sessions Judge at Saugor, R. Drummond. Kishore's sister asserted that their father had been insane for twelve years prior to his death, and his elder brother stated that on one occasion Kishore had jumped into a river from which he had needed to be rescued. He had also beaten his wife a fortnight before the murder and as a result of this she had taken him to a 'mad Doctor' at Mowa Khera where she had left him for six days. Kishore's mother suggested that her husband had been insane and that her son 'was also not in right mind.' A neighbour who had undertaken to grow melons in partnership with Kishore recounted how he had ceased to work and 'behaved in an insane manner.'

There are obviously considerable problems with evidence of this kind. The process of gathering, translating and recording this information is obscure. There is also a need to be aware of the legal, medical and colonial discursive practices in which the record of the Indian voices was formed.[58] The agendas of the witnesses who wanted to give this testimony must also be considered. But what is clear is that the intervention of Indian lay witnesses was decisive in having Kishore classified by the British medical and legal authorities as insane at the time of his committing a criminal act. The medical officer was only moved to assert insanity when neighbours and relatives arrive to attest to it.

The importance of witness intervention is also evident in the case of Kulloo.[59] He was heard to say that he must 'avert the black day by burning the thatched houses'[60] and as a result he set out to fire the huts immediately adjacent to his own. Upon being taken into custody he was sent to the Civil Assistant Surgeon of Baitool, one Henry King. He notes in a letter to the Joint Magistrate when returning Kulloo to the Jail that 'with reference to a person named Kulloo, supposed to be a lunatic and under observation in the Jail Hospital for some days, I have the honor to inform you that his conduct has not been such as to justify my certifying his insanity or irresponsibility for his action.'[61] Even when Kulloo was sent back to Henry King after attempting to set fire to other prisoners the doctor maintained that he was 'unwilling to certify positively that he is so far irresponsible for his actions as to be an unfit object for punishment.'[62] In a deposition for the case King asserted of the defendant that 'his manner has been eccentric but not positively insane.'[63]

Despite these refusals of the medical officer to positively classify Kulloo as insane the defendant was acquitted on the ground of insanity at the time of the commission of the act. Such a verdict evidently surprised many at the time. The Government of the North-Western Provinces contacted the Sessions Judge who oversaw the case stating that 'it appears . . . desirable to the Lieutenant-Governor that the Government should be placed in possession of the evidence taken in proof of insanity.'[64]

This evidence comes in the form of a *Translation of evidence in the above case regarding the insanity of defendant as called for in the letter of the Sessions Judge (no. 626) Dated 8th November 1860*.[65] In this are reproduced in English the following witness statements:

Ragho, Lohar – Defendant constantly roves about like a lunatic, and does not work for his livelihood. About 20 days since, defendant attempted to set fire to Sewa's house, about 8 pm; I and Ramsuhaie caught him in the act. A little of the house was burnt. I don't know whether defendant is given to intoxicating drugs.

Dewar – Defendant's conduct is like a lunatic's; he sets people's houses on fire, and beats his household. Ramsahoie's and Bodee's houses were fired by him. I have seen him carrying about torches.

Ramsuhaie – Defendant roves about like a lunatic, but I imagine him to be only of a sulky and morose temperament not really mad. He set fire to Serva and Bugora's houses and also to Gunga Deen's house in Baitool; I and Raghoo saw him light Sewa's house with a torch. He has fired several people's houses.

Juddonath Suhaie, Jail Darogah – Submits an urzee on 2nd February 1860

that Hoosein Mohamed, prisoner, had reported that defendant had taken
the 'chiraj' from Barrack no. 3 and burnt him and keeps pulling his
clothes and won't allow him to sleep.
Hoosein Mohamed – States that defendant makes a row at night, and
tearing his clothes, dips them in oil and attempts to burn me. He burns
other prisoners and won't allow anyone to sleep.

That the first three witnesses knew that he roved about and did
no work suggests that they are neighbours as these opinions point
to prolonged observation of his habits. The weight of opinion amongst
his neighbours is that he very much acted in an insane manner. If
such evidence was not enough then Kulloo's behaviour had been
sufficiently disruptive to bring him to the notice of the jail authorities. Details of this behaviour are included alongside the opinion
of his neighbours in order to corroborate the opinion that he had
been acting insanely. These witness statements coupled with disruptive behaviour in an institution were sufficient to have resulted
in him being labelled as insane. This in turn lead to Kulloo being
acquitted on the assumption that his insanity was of sufficient
longstanding to have included the period when the attempted ar-
son of which he was accused took place. Therefore the significance
of this case is that the defendant was judged insane *despite* the
judgement of the British medical officer. The evidence of Indian
witnesses, of neighbours and jailors was held to be superior to the
judgement of the medical officer. The presence of Indian witnesses
in this case was not just decisive. It was the sole factor in the
positive classification of Kulloo as insane at the time of the crime.

It is an administrative anomaly that has preserved these details
as no other administration within British India chose to enter such
cases in the A proceedings during this period and the North Western Provinces only recorded cases where there may have been some
procedural irregularity. Even then they soon discontinued this practice.
So, with only a few examples of cases with full sets of papers available it is difficult to establish just how often criminal defendants
were declared insane at the time of the crime due to the intervention of lay witnesses as opposed to the testimony of British officers.

Even if it were possible to establish such a figure its meaning
would be obscured because of the difficulty of finding examples
where the opposite was the case. In other words it would be very
problematic to attempt to cite cases where the failure of a lay witness to intervene had resulted in someone who was mentally disturbed
at the time of his/her offence being sentenced as responsible for

the act. This would involve trying to diagnose from legal records symptoms of insanity in defendants who were not perceived to be mad at the time.

There is however, the odd tantalising suggestion that the failure of witnesses to testify meant that those who were insane at the time of their crime were processed through the judicial system with little attention paid to their state of mind. The following example at least hints that a medical officer believed that he had found such a case. Gokhall[66] was admitted to the Lucknow asylum from jail. Consider the opening statement of his case record: 'A prisoner – had been violent and struck someone was sentenced to 6 months imprisonment – it then appeared he was insane – no history of his case is obtainable'. As he was classified on the case note as 'a prisoner' upon reaching the asylum it would imply that he was still under sentence. In other words his insanity did not become clear at a point where it allowed him to be acquitted and it is likely then that he was already in prison serving his sentence when his symptoms were noticed. 'No history of his case is obtainable' is a stock phrase in the case notes implying that it had been impossible to study the aetiology of his disorder. This was because there were no relatives/friends available to answer questions as to his previous behaviour. The choice of 'it then appeared he was insane' is significant. When prisoners were adjudged to have become insane while in prison an entry on the case note like that of Sooraj Bullee was more common: 'This man was a life prisoner in the jail of Lucknow. It appears that during his imprisonment he became insane.'[67] This shows in the case of Sooraj Bullee that when the superintendent was able to clearly state that he thought insanity was a product of the prison he would go ahead and write it on the case note. The entry 'it then appeared he was insane' suggests therefore that the superintendent did not feel confident enough to say that the prisoner had become insane in prison. The way that the phrase is constructed implies that the man's condition was being noticed for the first time rather than appearing for the first time. In other words it may well be that his 'insane' behaviour was of longstanding rather than something that started while he was under sentence.

If this was so then Gokhall's case note reads as follows. Because there were no witnesses available to explain his sudden violent attack, Gokhall is churned through the criminal justice system as a relatively unimportant assault case. His was relatively unimportant as his case note reveals that he was classed as an 'aheer' and a 'labourer' and so was evidently of little significance to the British as he was low income and low status. He was sentenced to six months in prison. It is only once in prison and under the regular scrutiny of the authorities that the unsettled mental condition that Gokhall was suffering from all along was noticed and an 'insanity' diagnosis attached to him.

Of course there are other ways of interpreting this evidence and the very unimportance of such a figure to the British makes it unlikely that he appears elsewhere in the colonial records. Consequently further corroboration of his case is difficult. Nevertheless, it can be tempting to take this brief description as evidence of the importance of lay witnesses in the fate of a disordered criminal. In the earlier examples the lay witness was decisive in the legal process ending in a verdict that the defendant was insane at the time of the act. There is certainly the suggestion in this last example of Gokhall that the reverse could also be true. The lack of lay witnesses to draw the attention of the British authorities to the state of mind of a defendant could result in a disturbed offender being processed as perfectly sane and culpable.

Jail transfers

This final example of Gokhall points to another category of prisoner who ended up labelled a 'criminal lunatic' in British India. This was the prisoner who was considered sane enough to stand trial and who was convicted of the crime with which he/she was charged and was subsequently sentenced to a term in jail. However this prisoner was then transferred from the jail where he/she was serving the sentence to a lunatic asylum as he/she was classified as insane while in the prison. A similar category of 'criminal lunatic' existed in the carceral system in Victorian Britain and has been the subject of a number of studies.

In her study of those transferred from prison to asylum in Britain, Janet Saunders concludes that while 'prisons were designed to cope with some amount of difficult or unruly behaviour, and the Warwick case notes show that aberrant behaviour and other symptoms of possible mental breakdown might be dealt with for weeks by the prison medical officer before certification was turned to as a last resort . . . it was violent expression of mental "disorder" that was most likely to lead to the certification of a prisoner.'[68] Walker and McCabe point out that 'the transformation of prisoners into patients has never done more than relieve the gaols of the obviously disordered',[69] and that often the classification of a prisoner as 'lunatic' and his transfer had to be the result of circumstances where 'his behaviour might be sufficiently violent or bizarre to impress even the ignorant prison staff.'[70]

Violent behaviour was disruptive of jail discipline and as such prison managers sought to relieve themselves of those who refused to submit to jail discipline by sending them off to the asylum. Watson points out in an important study that it was not just the spectacularly disordered who were branded insane and transferred from jail to asylum. He emphasizes that 'there was a growing awareness of a category of mental abnormality that caused problems of management,'[71] a category labelled as 'the weak-minded.' Penal discipline in this period operated through a system of rewards and punishments, and the weak minded individual was deemed to be he/she who was unable to differentiate between the two. Indeed, Watson concludes that 'it is clear from contemporary sources that the original meaning of weakminded (as used in the prison) was literally "unfit for discipline" on grounds of mental incapacity.'[72] The prisoner who failed to react differently to punishment or reward, and indeed who often failed to react at all to either was unsuited to the modern prison system.

Quite simply then, what the weakminded prisoner had in common with the violently disruptive prisoner was the fact that he/she was a complication in the management strategies of the prison. The prison authorities therefore sought to be rid of such complications by attaching the label 'insane' to those who behaved in such ways which justified the removal of the troublesome prisoner from the system.

The inmates transferred from prison to the asylum as 'insane' in the Indian system similarly seem to fit into either the violent or the weakminded category. When the broader context of penal policy in British India is considered in this period it is easy to understand why such prisoners could and would be removed from prisons. The behaviour of patients would have to be gauged in terms of compatibility with the priorities of the Indian penal system. By the end of the 1860s financial goals were central to these priorities, as the Inspector General of Jails in Bengal boldly declared: 'The basis of the existing system of prison discipline in Bengal is remunerative industry as the best instrument of punishment and reform.'[73] He went on to make it clear that

> I am of opinion that remunerative industry is the basis of all real refor-
> mation of prisoners in a country where religious instruction is prohibited;
> that prisons ought to be and can be made self-supporting institutions
> and that from the introduction of a proper system the ultimate repay-
> ment to the state of the whole of the great cost now incurred for the
> maintenance of prisons in India may be expected.[74]

By 1867 Alipore Jail, the most developed of Bengal's prison/fac-
tories was making a net profit of Rs 250 000 and was able to afford
to import jute spinning machinery from Britain. Not that Bengal
was the only administration to prioritize financial aspects of the
penal system. In the Punjab the industrial system in the prisons
was able to produce carpets of sufficient quality by the end of the
1860s to find a market in England.[75]

Such priorities, and the development of sophisticated systems for
using convict labour in profitable pursuits had a number of critics
and was the cause of concern for some involved in penal management. Arthur Howell noted in 1868 that 'it would seem that in all
Presidencies, and especially in Bengal, the remunerative theory of
prison labor prevails to an extent which makes it very doubtful
whether the primary object of the sentence – punishment – is steadily
and systematically kept before the prisoner.'[76]

Sir George Couper, who was the head of the Oudh Jail Department and who claimed to have visited nearly every jail in the
North-Western Provinces while Under Secretary to that Government
worried that while the object of labour in jails ought to be to 'in-
spire the person who has to perform it with the feeling that if he
can once get over the period of imprisonment he will take care not
to incur the punishment again', in India this was far from the case.
The chief cause for this was, in his analysis, 'the desire to make
jail labour remunerative, that is, to make the jails as far as possible, self-supporting.'[77]

Nevertheless the fact that such concerns were still being voiced
throughout the 1870s[78] serves to emphasize the continued prioritiza-
tion of financial goals in the Indian penal system. Where prisoners
were likely to be difficult to fit into the systems of organized labour
which prevailed in Indian jails some method of disposing of them
was sought:

> As recommended by the Inspector-General of Prisons North Western
> Provinces, His Honor was pleased to sanction the release from the
> Lullutpore Jail of the prisoner Sooksah, who had been sentenced to two
> years' imprisonment for harbouring a dacoit on the grounds of mental
> imbecility, blindness and inability to undergo labor.[79]

This is not an example of a prisoner who was transferred from prison to the asylum. Rather it is an example of the authorities admitting that they had arbitrarily freed a prisoner whose various conditions utterly precluded the individual from contributing to the manufacturing processes of the prison. Although this course of action appears to have been unusual it is an extreme example of the system acting to weed out those who could not actively participate in prison industries. A far more common method of dealing with such prisoners was recorded in the Proceedings as follows: 'At the instance of the Inspector-General of Prisons North Western Provinces, His Honor was pleased to sanction the transfer to the Benares Lunatic Asylum of Gunput Chumar, a prisoner in the Benares Central Prison who was certified to have become insane.'[80] Where individuals seemed unable to comprehend simple instructions or concentrate long enough to achieve a task, or where they physically resisted being put to a task or were liable to an unpredictable outburst which would disrupt not only their work but that of others around them, they were likely to be tolerated for only so long. The most common route out of the prison for such prisoners was into the asylum.

There was a crucial component of the industrial system in Indian prisons which increased the chances of such reluctant or disruptive prisoners being noticed and weeded out. This was the granting of commission on the profits gained from prison industry to the Indian staff of jails. In 1875, when the wisdom of such a system was being questioned,[81] it emerged that all of the administrations in India had used the system, although by 1875 it had fallen out of favour in Bengal, Madras and Assam. The commission granted varied from 5 per cent in Burma to 20 per cent in Mysore and Coorg and was usually granted to the head of the Indian staff as an incentive for them to organize prisoners in remunerative occupations and to ensure that the inmates worked: 'As Jailors know that the amount of commission which they can earn depends on their individual exertion in the manufacture and actual sale of goods, they are interested in obtaining a good out turn of work.'[82] Indeed, an interesting variation on this system came to light in the report of the Inspector-General of Prisons in the North-Western Provinces:

I may remark at once that there is an essential difference between our practice and that which held in Bengal. In both cases 10% on net profits were allowed to be distributed, but while in Bengal the Jailor or Darogah got the whole of this commission, in these Provinces he receives only a percentage of its amount, the rest being divided up by the subjoined scale amongst other officials named.[83]

The list of 'officials named' included assistant jailors, warders, Darogahs and 'deserving prisoners.' This would mean that there were staff (and apparently in the NWP some inmates) in the jails in whose interest it was to ensure the smooth running of the convict work. It was in the interest of such members of the prison to notice individuals whose behaviour made them disruptive of profit making activities and to have them removed if they proved intractable.

Indeed, in addition to this layer of surveillance, a curious feature of the Indian penal system as it developed in the 1860s meant that the disruptive prisoner in certain District or Central Jails would have been routinely under the jurisdiction of the local superintendent of the lunatic asylum. Having the local Civil Surgeon take charge of the prison alongside his other duties was pioneered in the North-Western Provinces in 1862, where it was decided that 'Civil Surgeons, who generally remain many years at the same stations, have a great deal of spare time on their hands, and having to visit the Jail every day professionally, are obviously the right men to have charge of the prisoners and all matters connected with them.'[84]

This system of putting the Civil Surgeon in charge of the local District or Central Jail became standard procedure throughout British India (except in Madras) during the 1860s. There was a change of attitude towards this system at the end of the decade and it was decided at the Government of India level that 'the existing orders might be so far modified that where non-medical men, who are well suited to the responsible charge of a Central Prison, are available, they should be preferentially employed.'[85] However, in practice medical officers continued to be appointed to the charge of even the largest prisons throughout the 1870s. For example, in the Judicial Proceedings of the North-Western Provinces was the following entry: 'Notification published granting Dr Whishaw two month's privilege leave and appointing Dr A. Cameron, Civil Surgeon Bara Banki, to officiate as Superintendent Central Prison and District Jail Lucknow, during Dr Whishaw's absence.'[86] The Civil Surgeon at a major station like Lucknow would also have been the superintendent of the local lunatic asylum. He was expected to make regular visits to both the prisons and the asylum in his charge. This would have meant therefore that bizarre and disruptive behaviour in prison inmates would have as a matter of course been a subject of the scrutiny of the local mental health official.

The case note for Rajoosoa contains a number of these elements:

> Oct 1861. This man was tried for murder of his wife and sentenced to perpetual imprisonment. Shortly after when in Jail he showed marked symptoms of mental aberration, scarcely spoke, would not work. Continually whined, was restless + apparently uneasy but had no definite complaint – seldom appeared to sleep. I had him removed to Lunatic Asylum. He was always quiet, never turbulent, but could not be persuaded to do any work. Sometimes tried but had no *jee* for anything. Appetite poor – continually begged in a piteous tone to be released – his general health was never good.
>
> Sept. 1862. This man has been generally quiet and perfectly harmless – has for some time suffered from diarrhoea, looks anaemic + is falling off rapidly.
>
> Octr. He continued to decline + refused food – died 29th Oct. 1862.[87]

While never spectacularly disruptive, Rajoosoa's melancholic state of mind had ensured a passive resistance to any attempt to get him to work in the Jail. This had been observed by the Civil Surgeon while attending to his duties in the prison, and had prompted him to use his authority as superintendent of the prison to order the prisoner's removal to the asylum. There the Civil Surgeon had recorded on the case note the details of Rajoosoa's behaviour as he had observed it both in the prison and in the asylum. In this example then it is possible to see the importance of the medical officer's dual role as superintendent of the prison and the asylum. This is also an example of the removal of a patient who, like the examples given by Stephen Watson in his case study of English prisons, was deemed a management problem in penal institutions because of an apparent mental incapacity for the demands of prison discipline.

A shorter entry for Akhroo, is more to the point: '1861. Prisoner. Transferred from Lucknow Jail. He had been melancholic and indisposed to work – general health very bad – he suffered from diarrhoea and got gradually weaker and died 2nd Feb. 1862.'[88] Again the prisoner was not violent but his state of mind made him passively uncooperative when it came to putting him to work. As such he was a hindrance to the management strategies of Lucknow prison. This therefore lead to his transfer to the asylum.

The following details suggest that Meera Buksh, by virtue of unpredictable and violent behaviour, is an example of an inmate who had been difficult to fit into an organized system of regular prison labour. He was subsequently passed on by the jail to the asylum:

> 1862 Prisoner. Received from Lucknow by warrant and certificate of
> Civil Assistant Surgeon. On admission was violent and very troublesome.
> Occasionally in very high spirits and hummed marching tunes (he had
> formerly been a Bugler in some regiment in the Punjab).
> 1863 January. For several months there was no improvement in this
> man's condition. He was dirty + could with difficulty be compelled to
> wear decent clothing. He was very excitable + abusive – within the last
> month he has been much more quiet + rational + works regularly in the
> garden.
> Feb. Since last report has steadily improved. Appears now quite rational +
> conducts himself with propriety. Discharged + returned to Jail Feb. 10/63.[89]

Throughout the period for which case notes are available, there
are constantly examples where violence and excitability are central
to the case notes of prisoners received from prisons. In the case of
Seetul for example, that is all there is: '29 May 1865. A prisoner
lunatic, is occasionally violent. 17 March 1871. Died of diarrhoea.'[90]
Then there are cases such as Balgobind, whose case note opens
with the statement, 'prisoner under sect.379 IPC, sent in from the
Lucknow District Jail, is suffering from Acute Mania, is occasionally violent', followed by a periodic update to the effect that there
is 'no material improvement.'[91] Such cases are common even at
the end of the period contained in the surviving case books.

The case note of Mosst. Kudro provides an interesting insight.
Carrying with her a diagnosis of 'hysterical mania' the following
are the opening details of the account given of her in the files:
'7th August 1869. Prisoner under Sect.363 IPC. Not violent. This
woman is a prisoner lunatic, sent in by the Supt.Central Jail Lucknow,
is given to very lewd and immoral acts.'[92] This would seem to suggest that it was not just violence or 'weak intellect' that obstructed
the smooth-running of penal institutions. If this is an example of
a prisoner transferred because she caused disruption to the management of the prison, it is an example of overt female sexual
behaviour proving unmanageable in a Central Jail where contact
with male staff and prisoners would have been unavoidable.

The case notes then contain ample evidence to suggest that the
observations made by historians who examine English prisons are
broadly applicable to their Indian counterparts in this period. Quite
simply, prisoners were classified as insane for behaviour which was
disruptive to penal discipline in order to justify their transfer out
of that system. Indeed this process is more readily understandable
in a system such as that which prevailed in the jails of the 1860s
in British India. There the demands of, and structures associated
with, trying to generate marketable products through convict labour

would have militated against tolerance of disruptive behaviour in the jail. This would especially have been the case where the officer in charge of the prison was also the officer in charge of the asylum.

Gender

The last example above raises the issue of gender in British admissions to the asylum. The female proportion of the criminal lunatic population in British India as a whole was extremely small. Females made up between 15 per cent of the asylum criminal population in the Central Provinces to about 3 per cent in the Punjab at the end of the 1870s. These small numbers reflect the tiny female proportion of those incarcerated in prisons.[93]

Among the 18 case notes in the Lucknow collection which can definitely be identified as those of female criminal lunatics, it is possible to find 14 on which details of the crime committed are included. Of these 14, eight include details which definitely link the female criminal's incarceration to crimes that she had committed as a mother against her own children. Of the remaining examples another two suggest crimes committed against the children of others. Both Mosst. Kudro[94] and Mosst. Mooneeya[95] have Section 363 of the Indian Penal Code mentioned on their case notes. This is the punishment section related to Section 361 of the Code which deals with the crime of taking a minor from its lawful guardian.[96]

A typical case note for the women accused of crime against their own children reads as follows:

> Dalooie (f). Mania. 40. Hindoo. Beggar. 16 October/ 63.
> 16th October 1863. Prisoner. Sent in by Deputy Commissioner Roy Bareilly.
> 18th November 1865. There is no improvement whatever in this woman's state. She is a criminal lunatic, and was tried and acquitted under Section 394 of the Criminal Procedure Code, of the murder of her two children – with orders to be retained in the asylum during H.M. pleasure vide no. 148 of 15th July 1863 from Govt.India to C.C.
> 23 August 1866. To be retained in asylum by order of committee.
> 26th Decr. 1866. Having been acquitted by the Judicial Commissioner on the grounds of insanity recommended that a commission be appointed under clause 3, Sect.395.
> 8th Jany. 1868. Papers sent with letter 56 of 8th Jany 1868 to Judicial Commr.
> March 10 1868. At a meeting of the Standing Commission under clause 3 Sec.395 of the Criminal Procedure Code no. 350 Jan. 25th 1868 Oudh Govt.Gazette, Daloo was pronounced sane and fit to be discharged.[7]

The following example is interesting as it suggests that the beginning of 1868 was a clear-out period at the asylum:

Soordiah. Mania. 25. Mussl. Labour. 8 Augt/ 64.
8th August 1864. Prisoner. Sent in by Deputy Commr. of Fyzabad.
8th April 1865. This woman is a criminal lunatic, and is awaiting her trial for murder of her infant. She occasionally becomes quite sane but relapses to the same state, and is at present much the same as on admission.
23rd August 1866. She remains still insane.
26th Decr. 1867. Having been acquitted by Judicial Commr. on grounds of insanity, recommended that a commission be appointed under clause 3 sect.395.
March 10 1868. At a meeting of the Standing Commission under clause 3 Sec.395 no.350 Jan 25 1868 Oudh Govt.Gazette – Soodhia was pronounced sane + fit to be discharged.[98]

Despite their bureaucratic nature, the case notes do occasionally hint at the very real personal tragedies involved. Ramdioh was 'said to have become mad from jealousy, her husband having taken up with another woman – in a moment of frenzy she killed her child.'[99] Mosst.Doolia was 'tried for the murder of her child, was acquitted on the grounds of insanity. Has since tried to commit suicide by hanging herself.'[100] Not that all the cases were of murder. The word 'abortion' scribbled in a margin suggests that Phooljaria had attempted to terminate the life of the child she was carrying. She was a widow at the time.[101] Emamee Khanum had been caught in the act of 'selling or trying to sell her child.'[102]

It is significant that so many of the female criminal lunatics in the Lucknow asylum can definitely be associated with crimes involving children, and the majority of such cases are of crimes of mothers against their own offspring. This reflects the influence of British, and indeed European, cultural understandings of femininity and motherhood in the judicial and penal systems. This is familiar from studies done of infanticide cases in Britain.

Roger Smith, for instance, concludes that 'Victorians... felt that infanticidal women should be objects of mercy,'[103] and points to contemporary texts such as *Infanticide: Its Law, Prevalence, Prevention and History* published in 1862 which claimed that, 'indeed, it is unhappily true that, from whatever cause it may have arisen, infanticide is not looked upon in the same light as other murders... There is no crime that meets with so much sympathy, often of the most ill-judged kind.'[104] Nigel Walker provides a historical context, suggesting that instances from as early as the seventeenth century show that sympathy for infanticidal women had a long history. For example Lord Chief Justice Hale in 1668 advised a jury how to approach their decision about a mother in a case of child murder:

'if they found her under a phrenzy, tho' by reason of her late delivery and want of sleep, they should acquit her.'[105] He then shows how the nineteenth century produced similar advice from leading judges, Sir James Fitzjames Stephen concluded of cases involving murder soon after delivery that 'women in that condition do get the strongest symptoms of what amounts almost to temporary madness and . . . often hardly know what they are about, and will do things which they have no settled or deliberate intention whatever of doing.'[106]

These attitudes were based on two sets of beliefs. The first was the belief that motherhood and femininity were synonymous and that the woman's natural role and inclination was child-bearing and rearing. Roger Smith argues that this perception was so pervasive that although 'on the face of it, infanticide was the antithesis of nature: a mother's perverse rejection of her natural function would seem an outrage calling for the strongest possible retribution,'[107] so perverse did the rejection seem that it was assumed that only madness could explain it.

The second element was the view that the physical efforts associated with childbirth, indeed all of the physical processes associated with the female's reproductive capabilities, were debilitating and incapacitating. It was assumed that, 'beset by a biological life cycle that was deemed fraught with periods of instability – menstruation, pregnancy, childbirth, lactation – women were considered to go through periods of insanity which sometimes led to horrifying crimes against themselves, their children or their mates.'[108] Indeed, it seems that 'doctors agreed that the biological life cycle associated with reproduction caused "a profound modification of the blood" and hence left women open to periods of intense mental instability.'[109]

With such a prejudice so firmly entrenched in British, and indeed European, culture, it is no surprise to see it reappear in the British criminal justice system in India. This is especially so as the place of women in Indian cultures, widely regarded by the colonizers as simply 'the degradation of woman by Hinduism,'[110] was one of the issues that the British chose to focus their attention on in order to emphasize what they regarded as the morally superior nature of their civilization in comparison to the cultures of those they had colonized.

For these reasons, infanticide was a preoccupation of British social policy in parts of British India from the 1830s onwards and legislative approaches emphasized the sympathy for women inherent in the

colonial British legal system. Throughout the period of consulta-
tion which led to the Female Infanticide Act of 1870 the tone of
advice was in favour of 'making the head of the family responsible
for the practice.'[111] Some even wanted to see to it that 'the onus of
proof of innocence should be on the father, who was to be required to show that the child died a natural death.'[112] When the
Act[113] took effect sentencing policy is interesting. In Kanpur, for
example, 'two cases were proved in which the mother and grand-
mother were sentenced each to two years imprisonment, the father
of the child to five years and two accomplices to three years.'[114]
The apparently high incidence of infanticidal women among the
female criminal lunatic population in asylums in India reflects the
beliefs of the British males who operated the legal and penal systems.
They had the conviction that women were vulnerable to the impulses of their bodies, impulses that were linked to the female's
'natural' role as child bearers. These beliefs were a product of patriarchal cultural meta-narratives which had produced specific views
of the female's nature and role. Child murder was felt to be such a
perversion of these views that it was believed that they must reflect insanity.

Conclusion

> Gaol Bahar. Mania. Muss. Beggar. 50. 10 Jan '61.
>
> 1861 Janr. This old woman had lived for years in my compound where
> she considered she had a right to a house in consequence of having
> been attached to the family of a former resident. Is very restless + excit-
> able. Sings + cries alternately + often makes a frightful howling – busies
> herself with dusting about the grounds outside the house – is a kind of
> pensioner. Lately she has become very abusive and strikes the servants +
> children in the compound – breaks thin earthen vessels + in short has
> become so troublesome, noisy and destructive that after many threats I
> have felt myself obliged to shut her up.
>
> May. Since her admission is much subdued. Is very quiet + frequently
> petitions for release.
>
> December 4th 1865. Died of debility.[115]

Although she is not a member of one of the groups discussed in
this chapter it is worth mentioning Gaol Bahar at the beginning of
these concluding comments because of the essentially local character of the decisions made about her which resulted in her admission.
Simply, she was incarcerated because she was a personal irritant to
the superintendent of the asylum. She was a bossy old woman who
was attempting to assert the seniority in the household to which

she felt entitled by age and length of service. Ultimately however she was surplus to requirements. Her admission is difficult to explain in any but these terms, there were after all no meta-narrative pre-occupations with old women or those who threatened pottery. Her incarceration is explicable in the quintessentially local circum-stances of a British official's household and the inconvenience that one individual with the power of incarceration was put to by the behaviour of another.

This study of the British initiated admissions to the asylums of colonial India has developed two key themes then. First of all there was a range of meta-narratives operating in this period to define who the British intended to incarcerate in the lunatic institutions. These meta-narratives were linked to the anxieties of British govern-ment systems in general which had a long history of concerning themselves with vagrant individuals and communities. They were also linked to the specific experiences of the British in India, where the encounter with an alien and populous society which had proven capable in 1857 of unexpected and violent resistance had made the colonial government committed to greater control and surveil-lance of Indian communities. Indeed, as was suggested above other broader cultural considerations such as the gendered construction of feminity and motherhood may also have been operating to de-fine those to be admitted to the asylums as lunatic. Vagrants, the volatile, the infanticidal and the violent were the broad categories of person which the British intended to incarcerate in their asylums and which were born out of these meta-narratives.

Yet explaining the origins of the categories of person being ad-mitted to the asylums does not fully explain who was admitted to those asylums. This is where Gaol Bahar's case note is useful as it is a reminder of the second theme of this chapter which is the essentially local and contingent nature of the individual admission. While there may have been meta-narratives operating to define types to be admitted the actual fate of an individual who somehow came to fit one of these types seems often to have relied on localized factors. This was most clearly demonstrated in the section which dealt with 'criminal lunatics' where the availability of witnesses or the passing of a criminal sentence in a prison devoted to manufac-turing were the circumstances in which individuals were singled out of the prison population for incarceration in the asylums. How-ever, the examples in the 'non-criminal' case notes which show those who ended up in the asylum first being admitted to hospitals, poor houses or idiot wards or simply being passed from police post to police post also suggest that the process by which an individual came to be in the case notes was far from being a well-defined one and was likely to be the result of a series of local decisions and contingencies.

Quite simply then, the individuals who actually ended up in the lunatic asylums in this period did so not only because their circumstances put them within one of the broad classifications which had developed in colonial imaginations as a result of the broad anxieties of governing India. More importantly the circumstances of incarcerated individuals were such as to have drawn them to the attention of the local operators of the legal, penal and policing systems. These operators after all had their own aims and imperatives worked out from the logic and necessities of their own positions and beliefs and which often went above and beyond simply obeying the general governmental urge to incarcerate the violent and the vagrant. In other words not all who fell into the broad categories defined as problem groups by the British were incarcerated, and those who assert that in India 'admission came to be restricted to only those who were violent and constituted a threat to European society'[116] are inaccurate because of the breadth of the generalization. It was those individuals who fell within the problem group categories *and* whose individual circumstances brought them to the attention of the local operators of the disciplinary systems who actually ended up inside the asylums.

4
Disciplining Individuals: Treatment Regimes Inside 'Native-Only' Lunatic Asylums

Nineteenth-century asylum regimes

Writers who have considered the asylums established by the British for Indian patients tend to agree that these places were rudimentary lock-ups for those admitted. Shridhar Sharma christens the period from 1858 to 1906 the 'second phase of development' and concludes that 'the asylums then constructed were simply places of detention,'[1] pointing to 'the apathy and indifference on the part of the authorities at that time, to the needs of mental patients.'[2] The work of Waltraud Ernst, although mainly focused on the asylums in British India for European patients, comes to a similar conclusion. She characterizes these institutions by the middle of the nineteenth century as simply 'refuges or temporary receptacles.'[3]

If Sharma and Ernst are correct then it would appear that the asylums of nineteenth century India were unusual. First of all it would appear that their rudimentary function as places of detention contrasted with asylum regimes in other colonial contexts. Regino Paular, in looking at the treatment of Filipinos in the Philippines during Spanish colonial rule in the nineteenth century pointed to the export of European models of treatment. He concluded that 'during the latter part of the nineteenth century, the psycho-medical practice of observing, analyzing, and treating mentally-disturbed Ss in the Philippines had traceable aspects of European schools of thought (e.g. Psychoanalysis), particularly in the use of psychopathological terminologies and in the rudimentary application of the Catharsis method.'[4]

Similarly, Sally Swartz considered treatment regimes in the Valkenberg asylum in the Cape Colony and concluded:

> Care for the insane in the Cape asylums during the period 1891–1920 was governed by four principles, which together formed the basis of 'moral management': 'early' treatment, in 'insipient' stages of the illness; classification of patients according to race, gender, and class of disturbance, separating quiet, 'hopeful' and recovering cases from dangerous or disruptive ones; remedial occupation and recreation; and minimal resort to harsher forms of control such as mechanical restraint and seclusion.[5]

Indeed, if Sharma and Ernst's conclusions are accepted, it would also seem that the asylums in India in the nineteenth century would not fit the model of those developing in the West at the same time. Historians who have looked at asylums in Europe and America have identified detailed treatment programmes within the institutions. These programmes had two aims, the first was to bring the new admission's behaviour under the control of the agents of the asylum. The second was to begin reforming that behaviour, to 'actively... transform the lunatic, to remodel him into something approximating the bourgeois ideal of the rational individual.'[6]

The process of bringing the patient under the control of the asylum began with physical treatment. An example cited by Michel Foucault is 'hydrotherapy,' where the patient was doused or soaked for long periods of time with high-pressure hoses. The underlying rationale was that first 'madness will be punished in the asylum'[7] and Foucault asserted that 'the use of the shower became frankly juridical; the shower was the habitual punishment of the ordinary police tribunal that sat permanently at the asylum.'[8] Yanick Ripa's analysis of French asylums for women came to a similar conclusion about modes of therapy which involved coercion or restraint. She claims that they were simply acts of repressive violence dressed up in scientific garb which were designed to chastize the aberrant:

> Treatment or punishment? The two words were in practice so similar that doctors often used them interchangeably. The insane had to be punished for being abnormal, and treated to put them back on the right path. Hydrotherapy was the cornerstone of this repressive treatment.[9]

In Ireland, Mark Finnane found a similar state of affairs. He discovered that 'although a therapeutic rationale had been constructed for the bath, shower-bath and douche (throwing buckets of cold water over the patient), by the 1870s it was commonly considered that they had come to be used "solely for the maintenance of discipline"'.[10] He also shows how the 1860s and 1870s were a period when pharmacological treatment became a means by which patients were controlled.[11]

Indeed, Anne Digby shows how even an institute like the York Retreat would use the 'pharmacological straitjacket' despite being regarded as pioneering humane methods of therapy. She lists potassium bromide and chloral hydrate as the main sedatives in use from 1858 onwards and quotes a patient who considered the aim of the drugs to be to 'quench the poor sufferers into quietness.'[12] Quite simply, these drugs were being administered to achieve the short term disciplinary goals of silence and obedience in patients.

Alongside the attempt to cow the individual implicit in such physical techniques the patient was submitted to the methods of non-restraint and occupational therapy which were designed to transform his/her behaviour. Taken together these methods came to be known by asylum practitioners as the system of 'moral management.' Anne Digby explored the system of rewards and punishments which made up the non-restraint regime at the York Retreat in England. The patients were allowed to go about without physical restraint and were treated with kindness and respect in all dealings with the staff. The idea was that the patient was trusted to behave, and this trust was made desirable by linking it with patience and consideration for the patient. The patient would then develop a desire to justify this trust and subsequently to moderate his/her behaviour to meet the expectations of those treating him/her so well. Digby concludes that

> moral management was depicted to the patient as a two-way process that involved both the imposition of a 'moral discipline' by therapists and also the development of a 'self control' by the patient. Eventually, it was assumed that internal restraint would replace external restraint.[13]

Non-restraint was designed to get the patient to go beyond simply obeying commands by those in authority to a state where the patient commanded his/herself to behave in certain ways and was able at the same time to obey those commands. In other words they were internalizing the moral order of the asylum, an order which was constructed to reflect an idealized version of the social order outside of the walls of the asylum.

Other authors prefer to focus on work for patients in the asylums as a part of the procedures of reform. Michel Foucault concluded that occupational therapy strategies were similarly designed to re-form:

> In the asylum, work is deprived of any productive value; it is imposed
> only as a moral rule; a limitation of liberty, a submission to order, an
> engagement of responsibility, with the single aim of disalienating the
> mind lost in the excess of a liberty which physical constraint limits
> only in appearance.[14]

David Rothman looked at an American example, of the Pennsylvania Hospital. Rothman concludes that when it came to treatment,
'of all the activities, asylums prized labour the most, going to ex-
ceptional lengths to keep patients busy with manual tasks.'[15] Speaking
of the superintendent, a Thomas Kirkbride, Rothman says

> he encouraged his private patients to do any task; it did not matter
> whether they planted a garden, husked corn, made baskets or mattresses,
> cooked, sewed, washed, ironed, attended the furnace or cleaned up the
> grounds. Outdoor chores were probably most healthy and pleasant, but
> the critical thing was to keep at the job. This regimen, Kirkbride and
> his colleagues believed, inculcated regular habits, precisely the trait necess-
> ary for patients' recovery.[16]

Feminist scholars in particular emphasize the importance of work
in re-forming those deemed mentally ill, as having the patients
perform work considered proper to their gender reasserted the cultural expectations of their gender over the inmates. It was the very
refusal to submit to those expectations in the first place which these
scholars believe had occasioned their incarceration as mad. Elaine
Showalter studies the treatment of women deemed mad in England
and concludes that 'the asylum's program of "suitable occupations
and diversions" enforced habits of steadiness and self-discipline.'[17]
She contrasts male patients' work, in workshops or on asylum farms,
with tasks allotted for the female patients. These tended to consist
of cooking, cleaning, laundry and sewing, and Showalter asserts
that 'women's occupations were intended to reinforce conventional
sex-role behaviour.'[18] Yannick Ripa concurs with this from study of
French examples:

> Work then was the antidote to pride and ambition, and provided a form
> of social therapy which put every woman in her place. Working-class
> women returned to the work they had traditionally done – repetitive
> and poorly valued jobs like cleaning, washing and sewing.[19]

Taken together then these various studies and historians point to
a range of techniques within the asylum which were to be directed
at the patient. The initial approach was physical intimidation, where

violence, isolation or chemical treatment was used on the patient to assert the authority of the institution over the behaviour of the individual. After physical intimidation 'moral management' techniques, the non-restraint of patients and the putting of them to work, were employed to encourage the patient to develop the correct habits of obedience, industry and self-regulation. The aim of this complex of techniques and the inculcation of these habits was to 'impose in a universal form, a morality that will prevail from within upon those who are strangers to it.'[20]

The evidence in the rest of this chapter seems to suggest that the regimes in the asylums of India after 1857 resemble these programmes of therapy outlined for European institutions far more closely than Sharma and Ernst's dismissal of Indian asylums as no more than places of detention would allow for. After considering this evidence and their conclusions, the implications of the treatment regimes in the Indian asylum for studies of the colonial state as a whole will be examined.

Asylum regimes in India

> The Asylum, I am to remark, should not be merely a place where the insane may be comfortably confined, but a hospital for their treatment and cure.[21]

There is plenty of evidence that the British authorities were intent upon providing institutions in India in which those members of the local populations that they encountered and deemed to be mentally ill would receive treatment with the recovery from their illness as the ultimate goal. The superintendent at Bareilly for example admitted that it was his job to see to it that 'in the management of this asylum attention is given to the comfort of the patients as well as to the cure of the disease.'[22]

It was suggested in Chapter 1 that 'recovery' or 'cure' in the Indian insane to the eyes of the British was denoted by an exhibition of certain qualities in the individual linked to self-regulation and productivity or what have been described as 'the Victorian fetishes, of "discipline, "routine", and "order"'[23] and of course 'hard work.'[24] Throughout the British administration it was considered self-evident that the best way to set up institutions to effect that state was on the lines followed in the model establishments in the West. In the asylums themselves superintendents wrote 'as we have now a good working establishment, I hope that we shall be able to carry out still further improvements, and in time bring the Asylum as near to the English standard as the circumstances of the country admits.'[25] Those nearer the top of the colonial bureaucracy had a similar vision, recognising that

> everything that constitutes a remedial institution on the modern European footing has to be introduced and exercised for the first time. The classification of the insane, the regulation of their common social life under the cottage system, their recreation, their education, their cure, their employment in various descriptions of appropriate labour, all the processes of benevolence and science have to be studied and carried into effect.[26]

As such it is no surprise to see the virtues of non-restraint, gentle treatment and the reintroduction to labour being extolled in the asylum reports:

> Herein lies the foundation of the good management of a Lunatic Asylum for natives. The hope of release, avoidance of everything that might annoy or vex the patients, unremitting watching, and silent attention to their complaints and ramblings will gain perfect control over the noisiest and most troublesome. The unreal and often rude speech must be borne, because to attempt corrections or to be angry with them will only aggravate and destroy control over the patient.
>
> I believe that by scrupulous cleanliness, liberal diet, affording them means of recreation or occupation, and attention to all the functions of the body are the foundation of the medical treatment and moral management of lunatics.
>
> The insane are not slow in sagacity and the power of comprehending what is done for their good and thus will appreciate kindness.[27]

The way in which the British medical officers used the therapeutic regimes developed in nineteenth-century Europe to assert themselves and their agendas over the bodies and minds of those who came under their jurisdiction in the asylums will be explored by examining the two stages in the process of assertion: control and reform.

Controlling the Indian inmate

> It must not be supposed, because the labor of an asylum is rightly called voluntary, that the character of a Native, naturally indolent and now exalted by mania, or depressed by melancholy, is of necessity by admission to an Asylum, in a moment so transformed that industry becomes a pleasure to him. It is of the essence of his treatment that he be brought, by resolution of purpose and persistent effort, within the discipline of the place if he do not at once conform to it.[28]

The first task for the medical officer on being confronted by a new inmate was to establish authority over that individual and to ensure that his/her behaviour and body met a basic standard from which the procedures of reform could take place. The body was the first site to be prepared.

The body

> On a patient being brought to the asylum he or she is placed in a single room for two or three days, well washed, carefully fed, the state and condition of the excretions and secretions examined... where there is any obvious bodily disorder found to exist, appropriate medicines are prescribed for its removal....[29]

The body was to be ordered through the regulation of its functioning. As such cleanliness, nutrition and rest were imposed and the working of the body was closely observed. 'Every patient is daily bathed,'[30] insisted the superintendent at Cuttack while the superintendent at Dacca gave more detail of the process in his institution: 'The lunatics, both males and females, are bathed daily... The dirty and intractable patients are rubbed with khullee (mustard oil culee) made into a thin paste with water and then washed under the shower bath. This cleanses the skin and leaves it soft, and is better than soap which makes the skin dry... one of the day keepers is particularly set apart for the bathing duties.'[31] The suggestion that cleanliness was imposed on the patients comes through even more clearly in the assertion of the Surgeon-Major at Delhi. He stressed that

> cleanliness is enforced both as regards the wards, the grounds and the persons of the lunatics. Nothing can prevent entirely some of the most debased of the lunatics from being guilty of filthy actions, but they are cleaned and washed and all traces of pollution at once removed.[32]

Coercive measures were also used to ensure that a patient's reluctance to feed or be fed was overcome. The superintendent at Colaba reported in 1875 that

> there were 6 cases of refusal of food. One was of a very obstinate and protracted nature in a young Parsi suffering from acute mania; he had to be fed with the stomach pump regularly for about two months; he was in consequence very much reduced. One day he was accidentally given some beer, which had the desired effect, as he began to eat soon after of his own accord.[33]

Indeed, the administration of nutrition could be even more violent still: 'Tea was also given by injection through the rectum.'[34] In other words patients had no control over their own intake, their diet was determined by the colonial medical officer and the food was then forcibly administered if necessary.

The body was not just subjected to washing and feeding, it was also deliberately rested. Dr Wylie at Ahmedabad was frank in accounting for his use of certain drugs, 'Hydrate of Chloral ... is a useful addition to the available means of controlling insomnia.'[35] The medical officer in charge of the asylum at Moorshedabad mentioned 'the administration of Morphia to allay undue excitement and procure sleep'[36] and the superintendent at Madras noted that 'a little wine or arrack at bedtime induces a quiet sleep, and I do not consider the use of opiates desirable where simple means can be employed to effect the desired result.'[37]

It also appears that vaccination was forced on the bodies of many of those admitted to the asylums. David Arnold has demonstrated that vaccination in the prisons of India was an unashamed assertion of the colonial will as 'at a time when vaccination against smallpox still encountered strong resistance and evasion in India, it was compulsory for prisoners.'[38] Consider then John Murray at the asylum in Madras who mentioned that 'vaccination has been carefully attended to'[39] and Arthur Payne at the Calcutta institution who indicated that not much choice was given to the patients: 'Vaccination has been practised in every case.'[40] In the Bombay Presidency

> at Ahmedabad and Hyderabad all the inmates are protected; but although the other Superintendents make no mention of vaccination, the fact that there has not been a single case of small pox recorded from any of the asylums even during a period when that disease was exceptionally prevalent elsewhere, and even in their vicinity, would seem to point to the effectual measures of protection having been adopted by all.[41]

These processes of imposing the order of the asylums on the patients were all accompanied by close surveillance of the body in order to gauge its progress towards a certain standard. In his report of 1872 Dr Penny at the Delhi institution notes the importance of physiological surveillance, or what he calls 'carefully watching all the functions of the body.'[42] One way to give this surveillance a scientific and empirical footing was devised in the Madras Presidency:

In 1874 I ordered the introduction of the system of weighing the patients monthly. This has been attended with great advantages, as an inspection of the register at once attracts attention to any patient needing care on account of deterioration of general health, or who may require a change of diet.[43]

Central to the policy of the medical officers then was a range of strategies devoted to the patient's physical state. This could easily be seen as an act of benevolence or just good sense on the part of officials dealing with admissions who were often starving or ill: 'A very large proportion, however, of our patients require no other treatment than good feeding.'[44] Indeed, the emphasis on the physical may also simply reflect the theoretical limitations, mentioned in Chapter 1, of doctors whose stock in trade it was to deal with the body rather than the mind.

However, it is necessary to consider more extreme examples of the medical officer at the asylum asserting himself over the body of the Indian inmate in order to fully comprehend the project of the colonial in treating the patient's physique. Consider again the treatments meted out to the patients in the asylum of the Civil Surgeon of Rangoon which were mentioned in the introductory chapter:

The very obnoxious practice of masterbation [sic] which is the cause of insanity in many cases, and which aggravates the disease, is very common amongst the inmates of the asylum here. I have perplexed myself about the vice and in former years endeavoured to prevent it by blistering the penis with crotenal etc., but without effect, and various medicines were given in vain with the view of moderating or repressing the desire.

During the past year I have tried Dr Yellowless's mode of prevention very recently practiced in asylums at home, and so far as it has gone, I am very much satisfied with the result.

The suggestion was founded on the anatomical fact that the prepuce was anatomically necessary for the erection of the penis. Its anatomical use was to give a cover for the increased size of the organ. If you prevented the prepuce going to that use, you would make erections so painful that it would be practically impossible, and emissions therefore unlikely.

The operation is very simple: the prepuce at the very root of the glans is pierced with an ordinary silver needle, the ends of which are tied together.[45]

This is an overtly and explicitly disciplinary measure in the context of which the control assumed by the medical officers at the asylums over the feeding, the cleaning, the sleep, and the blood of the asylum patient can be better understood. The legitimate use of the Indian's body was being decided by the British officer. The Indian was being denied access to his/her personal physical experience of the world and was being prevented from using his/her own body to convey his/her own messages or satisfy individual desires. Quite simply the Indian inmate's body had been colonized and it was to be disciplined by the British medical officers through enforced cleanliness, feeding, sleep and a range of other painful interventions.

The order that the medical officers were imposing is evident in the description of recovery on the case note of Mukhsoodally Khan, who was admitted for mania and suffered an attack of fever:

> For several months past this man has improved in health, has been quiet + well conducted and assisted in the garden – he is stout and strong – all bodily functions properly performed + he does not appear to be labouring under any delusion. His relatives are anxious to remove him + I therefore, as he has been well for months, discharge him cured.[46]

There is no reason on a document on which information is contained about an individual who was thought to be suffering from mental disorder to include all that information about the man's physical condition unless it is considered significant evidence in connection with the decision to discharge. If it is significant evidence in connection with the decision to discharge then it must be because it is indicative of the man having achieved the condition desired by the asylum. In other words, the asylum was seeking to produce stout, strong and ordered bodies, the result of all that feeding, cleaning and chemical treating. Asylum medicine seems equally as disciplinary as the colonial medicine described elsewhere.[47] It functioned to drill and produce bodies that could prove useful in a colonial system.

The mind

The production of a disciplined body was not the only end to which the efforts of the asylum were directed. The behaviour of the patient, 'exalted by mania or depressed by melancholy' needed similarly to be brought within the discipline of the asylum and under the control of the superintendent before the more complex procedures of reform could be attempted. This imposition of control would consist of rousing or subduing the patient according to whether the patient was withdrawn and unenthusiastic or over-excited and animated.

Official policy in this period was to follow European theories of controlling the patient through kindness and coaxing. In 1877 it was written in an end of year report that the system adopted in the asylum is what is called the 'non-restraint' system, the object of which is the humane and enlightened curative treatment of the insane. As is well known, this system was inaugurated by Pinel and Esquirol in France and by Charlesworth, Hill and Connolly in England.[48]

Almost ten years earlier the elements of 'humane and enlightened' approaches were described by an asylum superintendent in the North-West Provinces: 'Harshness and violence form no part of the system; coercion is seldom if ever resorted to; and the inmates are managed and quieted entirely by kindness, firmness, order, regularity and occupation.'[49]

Despite this rhetoric though restraint and violence in a variety of forms were sanctioned by the medical officers in charge of the institutions. There were superintendents who simply ignored fashionable opinion and went ahead with mechanical restraint: 'When refractory patients are confined in these wards it is generally found necessary to secure them with strait waistcoats, as most of them are very destructive.'[50] Surgeon-Major Payne in Bengal was similarly dismissive of non-restraint although he was more concerned to justify his opinions:

> So much has been said and written of late years respecting the treatment of lunatics without personal restraint, and popular feeling has been so largely enlisted in its favour, that non-restraint has given its name to the modern system and has come to be an expression for every thing that is kind and humane, while all that savours of restraint is condemned in the popular mind as belonging to an age of barbarism ... It would seem however that the time has now come when it may be said, without fear of outside indignation, that personal restraint is good or bad in the absolute, precisely as it is good or bad in the individual subjected to it.[51]

He went on to describe 'fixing the maniac on a mattress, with a broad sheet covering his entire body' and 'a long canvas bag with a collar fitting loosely on the neck, sufficiently wide to prevent any active or dangerous movement of limbs ... this bag envelopes the whole person except the head, and its edges are made fast by strong tapes to the cot on which the mattress is placed.'[52]

Other officers decided to devise alternative ways of achieving control over the excited patient's behaviour and in effecting desired changes in the inmate's conduct. In the asylum at Colaba the superintendent exposed how medical officers could overcome the restrictions on restraint and devise acceptable ways of punishing errant behaviour in patients: 'No mechanical restraint is adopted in the treatment of violent or unruly patients. Such patients are placed in one of the dark, boarded cells, or merely shut up for a few hours in an ordinary room until the excitement subsides.'[53] In this example then exclusion and isolation rather than direct physical contact were adopted to chastise and frighten the inmate. Indeed this example from Colaba is particularly interesting as on the same page of the report the superintendent stated that 'I have no remarks to make on the criminal lunatics, excepting on one who is noted for effecting his escape from jails and once from the asylum. On this man's legs irons are kept.' It would seem that in certain cases where forcible restraint was used it was mentioned separately to the treatment regime. Elsewhere the system of exclusion and isolation was also used by medical officers as a means of asserting their authority over disruptive or undesirable behaviour. Surgeon-Major Fairweather for example revealed in the Punjab that 'restraint has seldom been resorted to and when necessary, nothing more has been done than to lock up a refractory lunatic for a few hours, or at most days, in a solitary cell until he has quieted down.'[54]

Indeed, medical officers had recourse to other strategies to temper and restrict the physical behaviour of the inmates. These strategies were available in chemical form. The superintendent at Calicut admitted that 'the treatment has consisted in subduing great mental excitement by large doses of bromide of potassium, hydrate of chloral, morphia, and lately tincture of digitalis has been tried.'[55] There was a similar enthusiasm for the pharmacological straitjacket elsewhere in the Indian asylum system; the doctor at Dullunda asylum near Calcutta for example reported that 'digitalis and hydrocyanic acid have been largely used in the treatment of maniacal phrenzy, and the hypodermic injection of morphia has at times appeared more powerful than either. The latter is indeed seldom without beneficial effect.'[56] Such procedures were the first steps that the British officers took in asserting control over the behaviour of the Indian patients. It was the medical men who were dictating acceptable behaviour and using various means of restraint to restrict the possible modes of expression available to the Indian patient. The next stage came when the medical officers attempted to punish or attack aberrant conduct through a series of shocks.

Consider the following case note:

> Lalooie. f. mania. Mussul. Dullal. 30. 6 March 1862.
> October. This woman was sent in by City Magistrate, stated to be her

first attack of insanity, but I had her as a Lunatic patient in the Jail Hospital three years ago before the establishment of the present asylum. She then suffered for months from acute mania.

On admission she was very violent + excited, would not wear clothes, tore everything to pieces + struck + bit every body approaching her. It was necessary to put her under restraint, a Blister was applied to the nape of her neck + sharp purgatives administered. Gradually the violence of the symptoms began to subside – she took to the spinning wheel + for the last two months has been well conducted + quite rational.

Discharged cured, October 21 1862.[57]

In the case of Lalooie the stages between the state of excitement and the states of passivity and obedience are restraint and then blistering and purging. A similar impact can be seen in the case of Mhiboobun: 'On admission was very sulky and refused her food. Afterwards became violent and tossed about her head and arms, blister was applied and aperient given. Since then has been quieter and takes her food well.'[58]

The techniques mentioned in these case notes did have medical justifications. Blistering could be defended as a 'counter-irritant' in the belief that active disease in one part of the body would draw away morbid action from the brain.[59] Purgatives or aperients were a means of controlling body fluid flows by forcing the opening of the bowels and inducing defecation. However the moment at which they were introduced in the case of Mhiboobun, only when she has become violent, suggests that the shock for the patient of being assaulted by a British medical officer by having him blister the neck and cause the patient to suddenly empty her bowels was being used as a tactic by the doctor to counter paroxysms of excitement. Pain and shame were weapons in the armoury of the asylum superintendent in confronting behaviour that he considered undesirable.

An excellent example of the medical officer's awareness of the efficacy of techniques with medical justification as disciplinary techniques comes from elsewhere in the colonial system. The Commissioner of Rawul Pindee summarized the case of the death of Mir Baz in a letter to the Punjab Government:

Dr Lyons caused an enema to be administered in his own presence to a Pathan prisoner, who pleaded epileptic fits as a reason for not working. It may be assumed that the man was a malingerer, and that he had not had any such fits. Dr Lyons evidently considered the man to be shamming, and he adopted the enema, knowing it to be the most hateful infliction to a Pathan as a punishment and means of curing him of malingering. The man died three days after.[60]

The enquiry into this death conducted by the Government of the Punjab revealed further facts. It had taken two members of staff, the Native Doctor and the Medical Dresser, to administer the enema: 'The instrument used was Read's patent enema . . . the place where the enema was administered was the open yard in front of the solitary cells.'[61] This last detail caused a little unease even amongst the British officials of the period as a report noted that 'Dr Lyons appears further to have acted with impropriety and harshness in having the enema administered in public, instead of within the patient's cell, or in the hospital.'[62]

Indeed, when Dr Lyons himself was asked to report his actions he wrote a letter to the Assistant Commissioner of Rawul Pindee giving the following account:

> I considered the man was a malingerer, and applied the most disagreeable treatment appropriate for epilepsy; for this reason if the man be really ill the treatment will do him no harm; if he is malingering the treatment will still do him no harm, and be appropriate punishment. This is the orthodox rule for the treatment of malingering and has been followed by me in doubtful cases both in the Army Service as well as in this and other Jails. I ordered the man to have an injection of warm water to clear out his bowels . . . Yesterday morning I observed this man had been taken into hospital; he looked depressed and crest-fallen which I thought only natural after the treatment . . . I at once remembered that I had ordered an injection for this man about four days ago, which I am perfectly well aware is offensive to Puthans . . . the Native Doctor reported to me, at my house, that he had died about 6 o'clock, and that he did not think that he had died from illness, but from grief or shame.[63]

The enquiry decided that the post-mortem examination of Mir Baz revealed signs of peritonitis in the gut and that the enema was not likely to have been the cause of death. However, what this set of correspondence does prove is that there were certainly medical officers who were not simply aware of the disciplinary possibilities of medical therapies at their disposal, but that there were medical officers who were happy to use those therapies as overtly punitive measures. Dr Lyons' intention in ordering the enema was *solely* disciplinary as he did not even consider Mir Baz to be ill and indeed exhibited a certain satisfaction at having rendered the prisoner depressed and crest fallen. The public administration of the enema was designed to shame the individual and of course to inflict discomfort or even pain as a sharp rebuke to the patient's behaviour (that Mir Baz suffered physically during his ordeal is attested to in the evidence of Motee Singh, the Native Doctor, who pointed out that he vomited while the enema was being pumped in). Quite simply, this is a clear example of a Civil Surgeon, of which many were asylum superintendents, admitting that he had gladly used a medical procedure as a disciplinary technique and that it was certainly not the first time that he had done so. That this came to light at all was only down to that fact that the victim had died in this instance.

The case of Mir Baz is not just useful in providing context for the strategies of the medical officer in the asylum as it also demonstrates that medical officers were not simply concerned to calm excited individuals but also to invigorate the inactive or work shy. In asylum practice this meant dealing with those diagnosed as suffering from dementia. 'Much active exertion has accordingly been displayed by the staff and attendants in endeavouring to rouse the listless and apathetic,'[64] declared one superintendent, while another recounted some of the details of the process of 'active exertion:' 'A strong water douche, by means of the hose of the small hand fire-engine pump, was tried in two cases with success in rousing the dormant senses.'[65] Whether the patients were violent and demonstrative or feeble and distracted the medical officer would attempt to control and manipulate their behaviour through a series of assaults on their minds and bodies. These were designed to shake and shock them from their own ways of interacting with the world and make them more amenable to the reforming programmes of the institution. As one medical officer put it, his techniques were designed, 'to afford in fact any means of escaping from themselves for ever so brief a period, and turn the current of their thoughts into a more natural and healthy channel.'[66]

George Smith, writing in the *Annual Report on the Three Lunatic Asylums in the Madras Presidency* in 1877, excused the use of such measures by reference to the experts:

> Even the humane Pinel did not hesitate to resort to coercive measures and the experience of men of very high authority in this department of practical medicine, have put on record many cases to show that turbulent lunatics have often been made to act in a becoming manner by treatment which assumed a more or less penal character.[67]

Bizarrely, such a passage anticipates, almost exactly, the conclusions of Michel Foucault who wrote of the 'paradoxes of Pinel's "philanthropic" and "liberating" enterprise, this conversion of medicine into justice, of therapeutics into repression.'[68] While the seton and the blister, morphine and solitary confinement, the bag and the strap-down bed may have had medical justifications there is plenty of evidence that suggests that they were used as disciplinary measures. In other words the medical officers who used such measures had disciplinary intentions and the desired net effect of these measures was to punish that which they considered aberrant and ultimately to control the behaviour of those that the British encountered as insanes in the asylums. Indeed, examples like that of Maraie Singh who when 'a seton was put into his neck, he whined like a baby + cried,'[69] shows that such measures were certainly experienced as if they were punishments.[70]

Reforming the Indian inmate

Having gained control of the inmate the next problem for the super-intendent was how to get the patient to 'recover', that is, as was mentioned above, how to make of the patient an ordered, productive individual.

A potent indication of the ambitions of the asylum superintend-ents is in their conceptualization of the asylum and the inmate. Dr Payne in Bengal conceived of the recovering patient as develop-ing like a child:

> Practically the simplest and most rational plan is to endeavour to revive the brain from decay by imitating the course of nature in its original growth. Habits and associations are the soil in which the ideas of child-hood first spring up and in proportion to the care with which the former are regulated will be the soundness of the latter. It is through the disci-pline and exercise of the body that this end is achieved, and the organic functions of the brain developed, on the perfection of which, after bodily maturity the growth of understanding begins . . . the damaged organ is the last that should be laid under forced requisition during disorder. If this be done there is danger of imitating the well known results of urg-ing the education of children prematurely.[71]

In a related vein, Dr Wylie at Ahmedabad liked to think of the asylum as a 'well-regulated household' in that 'discipline and order are successfully maintained under a homely system of kindness, blended with firmness as occasion may demand; and, as a rule, the asylum is ordinarily as quiet and orderly as a well-regulated house-hold.'[72] The asylum was conceived of as a 'home' and those in it a family in which the patients were the 'children' and the colonial representative the 'father.'[73] This construction of the Indian patient is significant because of the colonial setting of the asylum where the 'native' was often construed as a child in relation to the fully developed adult that was the Western man.[74] It is also a construction which is familiar from asylums in the European context, where there was 'the prevailing view of patients as being in a state of childhood dependence'[75] and 'everything at the Retreat is organized so that the insane are transformed into minors.'[76] Quite simply, this positioning of the Indian patients in a relationship of tutelage to the colonial officer in the asylum reports demonstrates the superintendent's perception of his duty. He is not simply a jailor for the patients under his control. Rather he considers himself father-like in as much as he sees it as his role to mould, form and educate those under his control. Having established in their own minds the correct relationship in the asylum between the colonial medical officer and the patient, the medical officers developed a regime to facilitate 'recovery' in the patient based on the performance of productive tasks.

Work was central to the asylum regime and the inmates were put to a range of tasks in the asylums of India, from attending to farms established within the asylum walls, to performing maintenance jobs around the asylum and even to participating in cottage industry processes such as spinning and weaving. Dr Holmsted insisted that 'our chief means of cure is labour: if we can persuade a lunatic to labour, we have hopes of him.'[77] Through exposure to work it was thought the Indian inmates would become familiar with what were described above as the 'Victorian fetishes' or what one of the superintendents in the Bombay Presidency called 'such wholesome influences as obedience, regularity, forbearance, mutual assistance, diligence and industry.'[78] In submitting the patients to labour, 'none are allowed to be idle,'[79] insisted the superintendent at Delhi, the medical officers hoped to effect the 'recovery' of the patients, that is to train them to be ordered and productive individuals.

The asylum reports also indicate that 'improvement' and 'recovery' in a patient were only recognized by the British medical officers when the patient began to work. One medical officer asserted that

all the Insanes are encouraged to engage in work as much as possible and they generally do so willingly. On first admission many sit idle but the force of example induces them speedily to join in assisting their brother unfortunates. It is indeed one of the first marked symptoms of improvement when, from sitting in an idle, listless, unobservant mood, they betake themselves to work.[80]

The superintendent at Hyderabad went further than this, stating that 'nothing looks so hopeful as regards recovery as getting them to work.'[81]

In this way work was central to the modes of treating the Indian inmate as it became both the means and the measure of 'recovery' in the patient. The British wanted patients to be re-formed into useful and productive individuals by learning the virtues of obedience, regularity, forbearance and so on through constant work. The medical officers also used that constant work as an indicator of a patient's 'recovery' in as much as the individual's progress towards the re-formed, 'recovered' state was signified by the frequency with which work was undertaken.

Crucially though the superintendents hoped to do more than have the patient submit to their work regimes. The fantasy was that the patient would be, in the words of the superintendent of Dullunda mentioned above, 'so transformed that industry becomes a pleasure to him.'[82] This fantasy is expressed elsewhere, John Balfour the Inspector General of Hospitals in the Dinapore Circle deciding that 'I need only add that not only should there be nothing penal in the work undertaken, but the patients should learn to look on it as a privilege.'[83] It can also be detected in asylum reports which produce images of the patients 'singing blithely at their task,'[84] or which exclaim: 'I must say I never saw a more happy or contented looking set of lunatics; they work both in the gardens and at the looms with pleasure to themselves.'[85] To this end

> compulsory efforts and punishment for not working have been studiously avoided; at the same time every inducement by humouring their fancies, and granting them some coveted indulgence in diet, extras etc. have been employed so as to form a habit; sometimes, when other means have failed, they have been kept with the working party unemployed, and have of themselves taken to work from seeing others employed.[86]

In other words the patients were expected not to have to be compelled to work but to wish to work and to learn to want to work. This was to be achieved through the tactics of peer pressure and the offering of incentives. The British hoped to train in the asylums workers able to motivate themselves to be productive and efficient. The ultimate aim was a *self*-disciplined Indian.

Yet systems of labour were designed to do more than simply take those Indians incarcerated in the institution and turn them into willing workers. The allocation of tasks by gender in the asylum underlines this. At Hyderabad in 1875 Dr Holmsted summarized that 'our chief work is employment in the garden for males, and for females grinding the corn required for the asylum,'[87] whereas in the previous year he had included more detail:

> The women grind all the grain required in the asylum, they leep and clean their own quarters, fetch their drinking water etc.; the men are employed in cultivation, making drains, turning water-wheels, attending bullocks, levelling ground, working in the cook-room, brick making.[88]

Similarly, at Delhi, 'no manufactures have been attempted, but the males have been employed in gardening, in keeping the ridges and walks neat and trim, and in any other light labour they could be induced to turn their hands to. The women do a little spinning of cotton thread.'[89] A gendered division of labour was being enforced in the asylums by the medical officers. The emphasis was on women performing domestic tasks and men executing outdoor work involving agriculture and rudimentary construction.

It is also interesting to speculate that the types of work that each gender was expected to perform reflects an Orientalist image of Indian society, an image Ronald Inden has christened 'Village India.' He describes this as the British conviction that India was a society of small, independent, agricultural units where 'each village was an inner world, a traditional organic community, self-sufficient in its economy, patriarchal in its governance . . . a natural, organic and stable community of subsisting peasants.'[90] It could be then that the British were attempting not simply to re-form those they deemed mad in Indian society into productive individuals, but into types which were consistent with a colonial construction of pastoral harmony.

What is certain though is that the gendered division of labour was intended to reinforce sex identities that the British thought proper. This is an idea familiar from the earlier discussion of asylum regimes in Europe. Indeed, other features of the asylum regime in India served to emphasize gender distinction. It was a matter of course that women's wards were separated from the male ones, as emphasized at Poona where

> the construction of the asylum provides for the complete separation of the female patients in a distinct ward. Three other compartments, communicating with the central hall or keeper's room, are set aside, one for criminals, another for cases of amentia and dementia, and the third is occupied by the stationary and generally quiet class.[91]

Surgeon-Major Taylor at Delhi revealed a further practice that emphasized sexual difference: 'The diet scale is the same as it was last year. I think that the women should have more food. I recommended last year that they should have the same quantity as the males.'[92] Dietary practices in the asylum also represented British ideas about what India was and what it should be in other ways. The superintendent at Dacca referred to 'cooking, which is carefully done: lunatics assist in both the Hindoo and Mussulman cookrooms,'[93] and Surgeon-Major Niven at Colaba pointed out that

> the 1st class includes Europeans and Eurasians, and the nature of the diet is the same as that supplied in European regimental hospitals; the 2nd class includes Parsees, native Christians of all sorts, mixed races and a few non-descript people who are fond of changing their character, and wish to be a Christian one day and a native another; the 3rd class consists of Hindus and Mahomedans, and the diet is composed of flour, rice and dhall, and a small quantity of meat and vegetables; the diet of the 2nd class contains baker's bread, tea and sugar, milk and meat, as well as rice and dhall. The native Christians and Parsees are very fond of tea, and it would amount almost to an act of cruelty to deprive them of that article of diet.[94]

In other words the asylum was also arranged to reproduce the British belief in the separateness of the races and in some cases even of the Hindu and Muslim communities and to emphasize to the inmates of the asylum that observance of those divisions ought to be maintained. What is especially intriguing about the above passage is the suggestion that while in some asylums there was a separation of Hindu and Muslim diets in Colaba there was not and indeed meat was administered to all. If this was the case then it seems that the superintendent's conviction that he ought to be turning out healthy physical specimens, a state which he considered to be dependent on the inclusion of meat in the diet, had meant that he attempted to impose such a diet on those Indians who may well never have experienced meat and who could have had cultural and religious reasons for not wishing to do so.

Overall then, the asylum treatment regime, and work especially, was devised not simply to turn out productive individuals but certain types of people. Asylum design enforced gender divisions and communal divisions (see Figure 4.2 where the plan separates the male and female sleeping areas and medical facilities and Hindu and Muslim sleeping areas and kitchens).[95] The asylums were fostered environments where those deemed insane by the British could

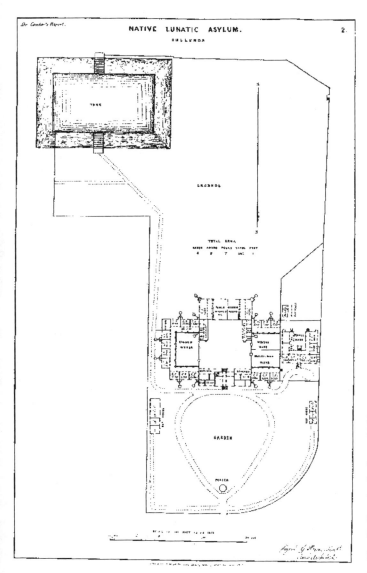

Figure 4.2 The Dullunda Asylum 1858

Source: Attachment in 'Reports on the Asylums for European and Native Insane Patients at Bhowanipore and Dullunda for 1856 and 1857', in *Selections from the Records of the Government of Bengal* no. XXVIII.

learn the roles that the British wanted all Indians to play. The asylum's population was to be productive and ordered, divided into neat religious communities and operating a gendered division of labour where the men worked at cultivation and the skills necessary for village self-sufficiency and the women tended to the domestic requirements of the men. These British fantasies, of what India was and what it ought to be, were built into the asylum treatment regime.

This is not to say that the reform of those Indians in the asylums was the only function of the treatment regimes in the asylum. Some superintendents had other ambitions for their schemes:

> Garden labour, soorrkee making, gunny weaving, twine spinning and stone breaking have all their special uses and are indispensable ... but without interfering materially with the progress of these, the labor of those patients who can exercise skill and judgement may, with advantage be diverted into more productive channels. With this object I propose to purchase, as the funds admit, some screw oil presses to be accomodated in the shed ... once obtained and in full work there is every reason to believe that they will contribute largely towards making the Institution self-supporting.[96]

This idea that the labour of the inmates should be remunerative and contribute towards the cost of running the asylum was formalized in the tables which had to be returned with the annual reports, so that the superintendents included comments in their narratives like the following:

> Statement No. 10 – This statement shows the profits of the labour of the lunatics which amount to Rs 781-9-4 for the year. As soon as I came here I introduced the manufacture of bon mooj matting in the Asylum, and during the six months the lunatics have worked at it they have made by this alone a clear profit of Rs 220-3-3.[97]

Indeed, if not engaged in industrial tasks the potential of the asylum population as a source of cheap labour was quickly realized. The superintendent at the asylum in Colaba recounted how 'a shed for the fire engine was found to be much wanted and an estimate for its erection was procured from the Executive Engineer amounting to about Rs 400. This was thought too much and the Deputy Surgeon-General suggested that the shed should be erected by the lunatics. The materials were therefore purchased at a cost of Rs 59-5-9 and the work commenced; and when it was finished the shed was valued by the Executive Engineer at Rs 149.'[98]

In fact, the systems of labour may well have had other objectives

still, such as sedation and control, as hinted at by the superintendent at Bareilly:

> I find that when the insanes are kept unemployed all day they become
> fretful and troublesome, and pass restless and noisy nights; but if their
> minds and bodies are occupied during the day, be the labor ever so
> slight, they appear to enjoy better health, and generally sleep soundly
> at night.[99]

The systems of labour in the asylums also had their pragmatic
side then in generating income for the asylums to offset the cost
to the Government of India of maintaining the institutions or acting to quieten the patients through fatigue.

Conclusion

This British vision of India and the way that the colonizers conceived of their project there have been summed up by Arjun
Appadurai. He concludes that for the British 'the project of reform
involved cleaning up the sleazy, flabby, frail, feminine, obsequious
bodies of natives into clean, virile, muscular, moral and loyal bodies
that could be moved into the subjectivities proper to colonialism.'[100]
It was this fantasy that was written into the case note narratives
explored in Chapter 1. It is this fantasy that also explains the complex systems of treatment devised by the British in the asylums of
British India after 1858. The asylum was one of the few sites where
the British had access to a population of a manageable enough size
to live out the fantasy of reforming the Indian.

The satisfaction of Dr Payne at the Dullunda asylum in mentioning that 'I have seen, and do daily see hopeless idiots rendered
useful by application to such work,'[101] is the satisfaction of a man
who is witnessing his regime producing the desired effect or in the
words of Appadurai the subjectivity proper to colonialism. This was
the Indian who was strong enough to work, who was productive
in work and who was self-disciplined enough to work. The attention paid to the bodies of the patients in the asylums reflects the
fantasy of re-forming the Indian body so that it would be strong
and fit to labour. The processes of first cowing and then transforming the Indian's mind through kindness, work and rewards were
aimed at producing in the ordered Indian a desire to be productive
of his/her own accord. Indeed the details of the regime, the dividing
of the patients by gender, race and religion shows that that asylum

regime was intended to do more than achieve the broad objective of providing useful or productive members of society. The strategies were intended to create subjectivities which would fit into the society that the British imagined or wanted India to be. This society was to be pastoral, gendered, and fissured along communal lines.

In examining the range of techniques and objectives involved in these treatment regimes it is difficult to agree with Shridhar Sharma's assessment of the asylums established under the British after 1858 as 'simply places of detention,'[102] characterized by 'the apathy and indifference on the part of the authorities.'[103] Indeed it is worth pointing out that these asylums were not unique in the British system as sites where the British acted to transform individual Indians. Gautam Chatterjee has argued in the case of the institution for juvenile offenders that it also 'provided an opportunity to intervene and restructure juvenile minds'[104] while elsewhere it has been concluded of the British penal colonies serving India that, 'one of the main objectives of sending a convict to the penal settlement of Andamans was to provide opportunities to a convict to reform himself.'[105]

Yet the evidence of the treatment regimes devised by British superintendents in the asylums can do more than simply dispute Sharma's account of institutions set up for those amongst the Indian population considered 'insane.' It can be used to reflect on the nature of the colonial state itself. It would plainly be nonsensical to see the asylum in British India as part of a coherent system of social control as Foucauldians see the asylum in Europe:

> A mechanized, regulated, and impersonal social system requires a high degree of conformity, and all the major institutions reflected the effort to render individuals obedient and productive with a minimum of violence and expense. Soldiers, children, workers, patients, and criminals were all subjected to a disciplinary system that attempted to regulate their bodies and souls, and their time and activities. The demographic explosion had created new masses to be divided into groups, subdivided into ranks, assigned fixed spaces, held to a strict timetable, trained to perform according to a precise regimen, supervised, judged, examined and classified in the institutional records as cases. The process of hierarchical observation, normalizing judgement, and constant examination controlled the education of children, the training of soldiers and workers, and the care of patients.[106]

The asylum in British India was not part of a 'carceral archipelago.' The Indian population in this period was not typically in a school, factory, reformatory or hospital. It was not therefore being subjected to the society-wide process, described by Major-Poetzl above, in which individuals were the level at which power operated to produce the obedient and the efficient. Indeed certain authors have argued that even when Indians were incarcerated in an institution considered characteristic of modern government then power did not operate as it did in Europe. David Arnold for example concludes that in the jails of British India in the nineteenth century, 'the colonial authorities . . . abandoned any pretence at individualizing or reforming prisoners.'[107]

Indeed, in looking at certain colonial schemes in India in the second half of the nineteenth century it is possible to see government power operating in ways that were anything but individualizing. With legislation like the Criminal Tribes[108] or the Forestry[109] Acts of the 1870s the British demonstrated that they were content to attempt to control undesirable lifestyles through community-wide repression rather than individual reform.

It is possible then to agree to a certain extent with Megan Vaughan's conclusion that 'colonial power cannot be the power which Foucault is describing.'[110] She is the only writer on colonial medicine who has seriously contemplated the significance of the psycho-sciences when exploring the nature of government in colonial contexts. She uses evidence which includes her study of psychiatrists and psychiatric institutions in British Africa to conclude that, 'the extent to which colonialism and medical discourse as integral to it, created "subjects" as well as "objects" and thus operated through individual subjectivities is open to question . . . although a great deal of what I shall call "unitization" went on in colonial states, this is not the same as the creation of individual subjectivities.' This she uses to back up her assertion that, 'colonial states were hardly "modern states" for much of their short existence, and therefore they relied, especially in their early histories, on a large measure of "repressive" power.'[111] In other words her evidence of colonial medicine in Africa, some of which was drawn from her study of the psycho-sciences there, led her to speculate on the nature of colonial government itself. Her conclusion from this speculation was that colonial operations were not acting to create individual subjectivities. As such colonial operations, colonial government in fact, could not be described as 'modern' as the institutional effort to act at the level of the individual to render it productive and obedient is central to any definition of 'modern' government.

Yet this study of the asylum regime has examined a system where superintendents could declare that, 'it is my endeavour to make the treatment as individual as possible; and the peculiar idiosyncrasies of the various patients are separately considered, and their wants attended to accordingly.'[112] All of the elements of the psychiatric systems of nineteenth century 'moral management' systems which were very much part of the 'modern play of coercion over bodies, gestures and behavior,'[113] are evident in the schemes of the British superintendents of India. Quite simply then, in the asylums of colonial India it is possible to see 'modern' colonial operations as they provide clear instances of regimes operating in which power was seeking to create individual subjectivities. The intention was not just to detain or to punish but to produce, that is to produce obedient, productive and self-regulating persons. Megan Vaughan may well be correct in observing that 'colonial states were hardly "modern states" for much of their short existence.'[114] However, in the treatment regimes of the asylums of British India in this period it is possible to see where it was imagined that colonial states were 'modern' states and where it was forgotten that they were not.

It is not the same thing however to explore what the British imagined their asylums to function as and to see how they indeed functioned. The next two chapters consider the ways in which Indians acted to ignore, frustrate and to collaborate with the objectives and the systems of the British which have been explored in this and the previous chapter.

5
Indians into Asylums: Local Communities and the Medical Institution

Imperialist medicine promotes political control, social inequality and exploitation, but it also contains many contradictions. It promotes new forms of consciousness, social structure and political action.[1]

The asylums seem unlikely places for Indians to willingly incarcerate themselves, their relatives or members of their communities. As has already been demonstrated, these institutions were implicated in the systems of social control and in the fantasies of social reform which preoccupied the British government in India. Yet it appears from the Lucknow case notes that Indians very quickly began to admit themselves or their associates to the asylums once they were opened.

As James Paul points out in the extract quoted above, Western medicine may have been introduced into local societies with certain goals in mind but the impact of the techniques and institutions employed could often vary from that which had been intended by the colonial government. The reasons why Indians local to the asylums were admitting themselves and others from their society into the asylums will be explored in this chapter in order to contemplate this issue of the unanticipated consequences of establishing Western medical institutions.

It should be emphasized that the step of admitting oneself or someone from the family or community into the asylum would not have been a matter of routine for an Indian in this period simply for the reason that the lunatic asylum would have been such an unfamiliar environment. As Shridhar Sharma says, 'The establishment, segregation of lunatics in mental asylums, and their supervision were entirely of British conception.'[2] Indeed, Indian societies had their own complex and well-established mechanisms for reacting to individual psychic distress to which the British lunatic asylum was entirely unrelated. In considering Indian responses to mental disorder, Sudhir Kakar points out that

> like very few other people, Indians have long been involved in constructing explanatory techniques for its alleviation... there are the traditional physicians – the vaids of the Hindhu Ayurveda and Siddha systems and the hakim of the Islamic unani tradition – many of whom also practice what we today call 'psychological medicine'. In addition there are palmists, horoscope specialists, herbalists, diviners, sorcerers and a variety of shamans, whose therapeutic efforts combine elements from classical Indian astrology, medicine, alchemy and magic, with beliefs and practices from the folk and popular traditions. And then, of course, we have the ubiquitous sadhus, swamis, maharajs, babas, matas and bhagwans, who trace their lineage, in some fashion or other, to the mystical-spiritual traditions of Indian antiquity.[3]

There is no evidence of hospitals on the Western model existing for the insane in India before the British arrived. Places of detention for the psychotic existed in some Muslim societies in the Middle-East.[4] There may well have been the odd charitable institution in India before the British arrived, such as that founded in the reign of Mohammed Khilji in the fifteenth century which aimed at providing for the poor and the vagrant in India and in which many of those locally deemed mad would have ended up.[5] None of these would have resembled the British asylum though.

This can be seen by comparing the plan of the asylum in Chapter 4 with an account of spatial use in a healing temple near Bharatpur which catered for those considered to be behaving oddly by their local community. The asylum design emphasizes the separation of functions. In the asylum there were distinct spaces for sleeping in, for cooking in, for working and walking in and in which treatment would be dispensed for physical illness. In contrast, Sudhir Kakar's account of the healing temple shows how at any one moment there is a welter of activity all within the same space. 'Patients', their relatives and the priests eat, sleep, pray and exorcise all in the same courtyards which they share with local urchins and stray dogs.[6]

This spatial contrast reflects a more profound difference in the aims and approaches, indeed in the understanding of mental illness, between the culture from which the lunatic asylum emerged in early modern Western Europe and the cultures in which the local healers and temple practitioners developed in India. In Europe, by the nineteenth century, madness had come to be perceived as having 'a hold on Western culture which makes possible all contestation, as well as total contestation.'[7] The asylum was a specific response to this cultural perception, it was 'a religious domain without religion, a domain of pure morality, of ethical uniformity,'[8] to be used as 'an instrument of moral uniformity and of social denunciation.'[9]

In India, Kakar finds that 'the restoration of the lost harmony between the person and his group . . . was one of the primary aims of the healing endeavours in the local and folk traditions.'[10] To this end it is necessary to 'avoid isolating the individual',[11] and so 'beliefs about a mad-person's actions do not implicate the individual's self but instead focus on causes external to the individual, often supernatural ones.'[12] In Northern India, for example, '*peshi* ritual attempts to transform the patient's belief into a conviction that his bad traits and impulses are not within but without; that they are not his own but belong to the *bhuta*.'[13] Therapy is not an individual undertaking but a group practice: 'When a mad person is believed to have been possessed by a demon, the whole family, their relatives and neighbours, sometimes the whole village, join together to plan, carry out and pay for the appropriate exorcism ceremony.'[14] If a sacred institution is visited for treatment, the temple rituals will emphasize 'the involvement and the integration of the patient's relatives in the healing process.'[15]

These traditions contrast with the aims and processes of the lunatic asylum. Isolated from society behind the walls of the institution 'the insane were "treated" by being forced to recognize and accept responsibility for their guilt . . . the inmates were not merely observed and judged by others but were required to examine and judge themselves.'[16] The asylum was not 'a free realm of observation, diagnosis, and therapeutics; it is a juridical space where one is accused, judged and condemned, and from which one is never released except by the version of this trial in psychological depth – that is, by remorse.'[17] The lunatic asylum sought to impose a *moral* system on the patient through isolation and inducing guilt within the individual. The Indian approaches emphasized the need to reintegrate the individual with his/her *social* system, and as such avoided isolation of the individual and advocated group involvement in treatment. It is difficult to contest the view that 'in India, mental asylums were entirely a British conception.'[18]

The asylums which were established in British India were alien spaces because they used techniques based on conceptions of mental illness which were very different from those of the societies around the walls. Yet for all this there are case notes available at the Lucknow lunatic asylum which suggest that Indians were admitting themselves or members of their families and communities to this alien space. These cases will be looked at in three groups those who decided to admit themselves to the asylum, those who were admitted by others but were reclaimed from the institution and those who were abandoned by members of their families to the institution.

Self admissions

> Bhagooie. Dementia. Mussulman. Beggar. 45. 19 March 1861.
>
> Mar 1861. This woman had long been a vagrant beggar in Lucknow and was in the habit of sleeping under the archways in the Cheenie Bazaar. She was almost destitute of clothing, dirty and lousy – She came and herself begged for admission into the asylum – she is evidently a person of weak intellect – is also suffering from venereal disease.
>
> 1862. This woman improved very much in general health and habits by attention and kind treatment. Altho' evidently of weak intellect, she had a fair understanding of her position and on her husband being discovered, showed an anxiety to leave the Asylum and join him.
>
> She was discharged, cured. Sept. 21/ 1862.[19]

Women in north India occupy a very precarious position in society, as Roger and Patricia Jeffery have stated after their study of the contemporary situation: 'A key feature of the position of all women remains their dependence on men.'[20] They go on to show how in modern north India the woman is more likely to have left her natal village and to live her life in her affinal village after marriage. Her position and security there are derived from the presence of her husband.

If this was the case in the 1860s it is a useful context for exploring Bhagooie's experience. The story strongly suggests that she was abandoned by her spouse at a time when she would no longer have been valued as a member of the village community. Her position in the village would have been difficult for three sets of reasons. The first of course was that she was unlikely to be originally of that village and would have been a member by virtue of having moved there upon her marriage to a son of the village. However, that husband had now left her and as such she would have been perceived as an outsider. Indeed, because she was growing old the village would not have valued her as a source of reproductive or productive labour as her advancing years would have made her unlikely to bear more children and would have limited her ability to work. Abandoned by the justification for her being in the village, and no longer valued by her affinal community it is no surprise that she came to be separated out from the community whether through choice or through coercion.

Whichever was the case her fate as a single woman without access to a community was to take to begging, a harsh and distressing lifestyle which apparently caused her to become ill. Realising that she was ill and that her position was worsening she sought shelter in the nearby British institution which happened to be the lunatic asylum. The doctor admitted her as he saw her ill through neglect and diagnosed the jumbled thoughts of one who had suffered desertion, illness and starvation as 'weak intellect.'[21]

Once in this refuge, where she was fed and could rest unmolested, she quickly regained her health and her perspective. When the husband was found by the British authorities, whose policy it was to try and find the relatives of all harmless, wandering lunatics, she was eager to return to her 'normal' existence which she had never wished to desert in the first place. In her case then, the asylum can be seen to have been a place that she used to recover from a crisis in her life. She took advantage of it to regain her strength and to shelter from the harshness of an unexpected period as a vagrant:

> Bhugwan Deen. Mania. aheer. beggar. 40. 20 April '61
> 1861 April. This man is a beggar by profession and for some time has lived in the Ameenabad Bazaar. He of his own accord begged admission into the Asylum – He appears perfectly quiet and inoffensive – has a very vacant expression and countenance – never speaks unless spoken to – fancies that he is sovereign of the world – Doorgah ke Malik – and has large armies, palaces equipages etc. at his command.
> 1863. This poor creature continued very happy and contented in the Asylum, generally enjoying very good health – During the rains of 1863 he was several times affected with Diarrhoea which as often got well – During the cold weather he became dropsical, the Diarrhoea returned and he gradually sank and died 17th Dec 1863.[22]

Bhugwan Deen is another of the self-admissions who appears to have built the facilities of the British asylum into his survival strategies. He was advancing in years and had been on the streets in poverty long enough to become known as 'a beggar by profession.' Little wonder then that the regular meals and ordered existence within the British institution would have appeared an appealing prospect. In order to gain admission he shammed a little with a tale about imagining himself a member of royalty and having got inside he gave no trouble to anyone. Indeed he appears to have been quite content to wile away his days looking forward to his sleep and his food. There is every reason to suspect that he was shamming as there is no mention of his delusion again on the case note. This is unusual as other case notes reveal that the British medical officers keenly recorded the progress of their patient's delusions as and when they manifested themselves.[23] Indeed, it might also be pointed out that if he really did believe he was 'sovereign of the world' then it seems odd that he would choose somewhere as modest as the lunatic asylum as his residence. There is also evidence from another group of patients in the asylum that shamming to gain entry was an option when a period there was deemed desirable. This group is the prisoners admitted from the Jail to the asylum.

For a prisoner awaiting trial, feigned madness was a way of establishing a defence. If it was suspected that the defendant was mad at the time that the crime was committed, then he/she would be acquitted once sane enough to stand trial. It was in the interests of the accused to be sent to the asylum on, or soon after, the arrest to increase the chances that the insanity observed then would be linked to the circumstances of the crime. For the prisoner already tried and serving a long sentence, the asylum was attractive as it did not force its inmates to labour, whereas many of the prisons did.[24] In addition, small indulgences like tobacco or sweetmeats were allowed the patients while such luxuries were denied the prisoners. It seems that some did try to pretend to be insane for these reasons:

> Mongloo. amentia. 30. Hindoo. cultivator. 30 Augt .64. Prisoner.
> 1862 A Pasee [sic] – accused of Dacoitee + sent in for observation by Dr Lane, Offg D.C. as he feigned madness – Several of his gang have already been transported or sentenced. I could not detect any real insanity. He was very much on his guard not to betray himself, so I sent him back to the D.C. for trial.
> Discharged 6th September 1864.[25]

Not that all of the prisoners who tried to get themselves a place in the asylum rather than the prison failed. An interesting case occurred in the Central Provinces:

Only one man (Dina whose case was referred to in para. 3 of last year's report) was re-admitted into the Nagpur Asylum. The Superintendent, Doctor Brake, thus reports about him:

'This man was very intractable at the Nagpur Central Jail, dirty in his habits, full of antics, refusing to work and reported to be sleepless at nights, but no sooner was he received back into the asylum, than all symptoms of insanity disappeared; the man slept, ate and worked well and was frequently employed in supervising others, always assisting them in their several occupations. He remained till November 13th the day preceding the expiry of his sentence when he was made over to the Jail authorities for release as quite sane.'[26]

It can be inferred that his first period in the asylum had agreed with Dina as much as his second stay did otherwise the British would not have returned him to the prison in the first place in the belief that he was sane. However, having had a chance to compare the two regimes Dina seems to have quickly decided that the asylum was preferable. He therefore appears to have set out to behave in ways that he felt would get him transferred from the prison back into the asylum, behaviour he did not particularly enjoy putting on as he quickly abandoned it once back in his preferred institution. His strategy to get through his sentence in as comfortable a manner as possible worked out as a complete success as he managed to see out the remaining months of his time in the asylum rather than the prison.

Of course it is impossible to say for sure that those who appear to be feigning madness or were accused of having done so at the time were actually doing so. It must be said though that as either vagrants or prisoners life on the streets or in the jail could at some point have involved contact with or witnessing someone who was subsequently institutionalized as a lunatic. In other words there would have been opportunities for the beggar or the convict to observe what types of behaviour guaranteed admission into the asylum. If the need to gain admission arose, behaviour which would be perceived as insane could then have been simulated.

Bhugwan Deen and Bhagooie, and indeed the prisoners who feigned madness and like the beggars are examples of self-admission, seem to have been using the asylum as a sort of refuge. Simply, they incorporated the British institution into their strategies for survival. The same seems to be true of the other patients on whose case notes self-admission was explicitly noted such as Boata Shaw,[27] who 'applied himself for admission' and whiled away his days working in the garden until he died seven years later.

Indeed the British themselves fretted that their medical institutions were being used by Indians in such ways. In an article in 1877 printed in the *Indian Medical Gazette*, entitled 'Poor-Houses or Hospitals?' the editor thundered: 'It is not fair that dispensaries, and the medical profession at large, should have this duty of a Parish relief wholly put upon them.' He went on to describe a figure considered familiar at the dispensary by medical officers, a man

who is notoriously a professional beggar. Times are hard with him, and he has determined that it will be comfortable to pass the winter as a house patient. He accordingly arranges to be picked up by the police and carried thither as a 'destitute'.[28]

Certain members of the local community were actively incorporating local medical institutions into their survival strategies, colonizing the relatively sheltered space made available by the British to suit their needs and agendas. It should also be pointed out that there is no evidence that these patients were admitting themselves out of a desire for access to Western methods of therapy for mental health, or under the conviction that they were mentally ill and needed treatment: they were admitting themselves to make their lives safer and more comfortable.

Family and community admissions

As already stated the Indians admitted by their families or communities can roughly be divided in terms of their fate. There were those who were subjected to a short period in the institution by those around them while there were others who were abandoned to it altogether. Those who were reclaimed will be considered first:

Mooloowa. Mania ch. 22. Hindoo. Labour. 28 Sept/65.
29th Septr 1865. Sent to the asylum at the request of his Uncle Seeun Village Samgunpoor as they had no means of keeping him under control – is very violent and abusive.
1st Feby 1866. As bad as ever.
7th May 1866. Made over to his mother by order of the Visiting Committee.[29]

In this example, it seems that the 'control' sought by his family is unlikely to have been simply physical restraint. Various accounts show how Indians devised ways of restricting the physical freedom of those within their community without involving the British authorities. The Lucknow case notes have a couple of examples such as Deerumeere who was 'found wandering about the district with irons on his legs, put on by his relatives to keep him fast',[30] or Nundia who appears to have 'escaped from his home in chains where he had evidently confined for years.'[31] Other devices are mentioned in other sources. A witness in a murder case described the proceedings once the member of a neighbouring family started having fits of violent behaviour. 'Zalim was then put into the stocks by his brother. I never saw him out of them. He had his food whilst in the stocks, and answered the calls of nature in the same place.'[32] The District Superintendent of Police for the area described the stocks. 'They consisted of a piece of wood roughly fashioned by the relations themselves and did not belong to any outpost or station. The latter stocks have been entirely done away with for some time back.'[33]

In Mooloowa's case then, physical restraint was unlikely to have been the objective of the committal. Mooloowa was being punished. The idea of committing family members as a means of disciplining them is familiar from studies done of the place of the asylum in other societies:

A young slater's assistant, apparently living with his parents, was committed for threatening to cut his father's throat, having a razor, and 'delusions.' On admission he smelled of whiskey, seemed to be recovering from a drunken bout but was quite rational and coherent. A few days before, he said, he tried to separate his father and mother in a family quarrel; both were drunk. They subsequently swore informations against him, and in his words 'had him sent here to teach him a lesson.' A week after admission his father came to take him out on bail; questioned by the doctor, he corroborated the son's story. He 'moreover assured me that at no time did he consider his son insane, but that he thought it would do him (the son) good to get a few days here.'[34]

Using such archival examples, Mark Finnane constructs the argument that in Ireland, during the same period as is being discussed here, 'the use of the asylum, or the threat of it, as an instrument of control in the family could be quite blatant.'[35] This conclusion would seem applicable to the example of Radha, aged 25, who appears in the Lucknow case notes:

Radha. Mania. 25. Brahmin. Cult. 1 Feby/65.
1st Feby 1865. Sent in by City Magistrate of Lucknow.
22nd April 1865. This man was brought by his brother for confinement, he was found very difficult to manage at home – constantly running about his village abusing the women. No improvement since admission.
Septr 1865. Made over to his friends at their request.[36]

He was obviously embarrassing his relatives with his behaviour towards the womenfolk where he lived and evidently refusing to obey his family's wish that he refrain from such behaviour. As such certain members of the family had decided to punish him by severing him from his community and admitting him into the strange institution. It was only meant to be a punishment though as he was not abandoned, being collected from the asylum again a few months later.

The step of committing to an asylum was not done simply to have the person restrained then, the Indian community could do this without involving the British. To remove the errant member from his kin-group into an unfamiliar institution where he was exposed to an alien regime was indeed a punishment as it denied the person access to the group for whom his behaviour was meant to have significance and isolated him from the people his actions were meant to influence. For the family, or the member of the family who had taken the responsibility for the step, it was a way of asserting the authority of the status quo to which the disruptive behaviour had been a challenge.

It is interesting to note that most of the examples of Indians admitted by Indians for a short term are junior members of the family being committed by senior ones. Mooloowa quoted above was 22 years old and admitted by his uncle. Shew Dial was 28 years old and 'brought to the Asylum by his father who is a chowkidar in Lucknow.'[37] Kandhya was only 20 and was 'said to have attempted to fire his village and to have been so violent as to be uncontrollable by his brother.'[38] Clearly then, those within the family with power were exercising it to discipline those over whom their authority was held. However this was a punitive rather than a purgative exercise. The family or community was asserting its authority over a member who was considered to be transgressing its correct functioning but who as a young man was valuable enough as a source of labour and of status not to abandon.

If committal could be a disciplinary procedure, the admission of young women for 'puerperal mania' is intriguing. This was the name given in the nineteenth century to erratic behaviour in new mothers in the immediate post-partum period. In Victorian Britain, motherhood was constructed as the 'pure and almost sacred state'[39] of femininity. As such, many women who behaved in ways viewed as unfeminine in the post-partum period, be it flaunting their sexuality, threatening violence or expressing extreme emotion, were deemed to be acting in a deviant manner and were treated as lunatics.

In India childbirth is similarly given cultural meaning, although the text varies somewhat from the British example. Studies of contemporary India show that 'a new mother is unclean for five weeks. For all that time no one should eat food which she has cooked.'[40] She is considered embarrassing, 'her physiological processes are shameful, distasteful and striking evidence of her sexuality.'[41] It seems that the culture chastises her for her behaviour in childbirth by denying her access to her natal family for a specified period after the birth.

If this was the case in the 1860s then there appears to be an interesting convergence of cultures between the British medical officers at the asylum and the Indian men of the local communities. Both of these groups would have considered female behaviour in the period immediately after childbirth as potentially problematic. As such cases like that of Mosst. Goolaba are especially intriguing:

> Mosst. Goolaba. Puerperal Mania. 25. Hindoo. Labour. 15th June 1870. Certified by the Magistrate. Talks nonsense.
> 15th June 1870. Sent in by the Magistrate of Lucknow it is evidently a case of puerperal mania the woman has become mad after the birth of each child.
> 11th July. Admitted for treatment by order of the Committee.
> 5th Decr 1870. Discharged much improved and made over to her mother.[42]

There is very strong evidence here that her family was involved in her admission. It seems unlikely that she has been admitted to the asylum before as a previous admission was usually traced and remarked upon in the case notes.[43] The information that she has on other occasions behaved in a similar manner to that which she was exhibiting on admission is likely therefore to have come from someone who the superintendent would accept such information from in other words a member of her family who he would have found credible as a witness to her other births. That such a family exists for her is proven by the fact that her mother came to collect her. She was not noted as violent, which other records suggest would have been the case if she had been,[44] so it seems unlikely that she had been brought in by the police. The only misdemeanour noted is that she expressed herself in unfamiliar verbal formulations, that is she 'talks nonsense.' It is probable that the only people in a position to have noticed this and to have been in a position to inform the medical officer writing the case note would have been her family as it would not have been likely, especially in the post-partum period, that anyone else would have had access to her. In other words this looks very much as if it was a family admission.

The only clue that the case note offers as to what behaviour had warranted her admission to the asylum was that she 'talks nonsense'. This could be less a symptom of illness and more the key to explaining her admission. A refusal to talk in the prescribed manner, which is likely to have entailed, or been interpreted as entailing, a lack of respect for senior members of her family has been linked with the local understanding of childbirth as a time when the female is most in defiance of the norms established for her by the patriarchal culture and it has been decided that hers was a challenge to the established order of the family. She was therefore banished from that unit until such time as she again recognized the authority of that order. She was not abandoned though as she was valuable, being young enough to be productive and having proven to be reproductive. So she was taken back when 'Much improved', that is, when once more quiet and respectful, and after a lengthy enough time for her to have become dissociated from her sexualized period.

There are then reasons to believe that the involvement of families in the admission of junior members of the family to the alien space that was the British asylum seems in certain cases to have been a disciplinary measure. There is no evidence that these families and communities were admitting their members out of a desire for access to Western methods of treatment for mental health, or even in the belief that they were mentally ill and were in need of therapy. There is evidence that those admitted by their families or community members had been exhibiting behaviour which would have embarrassed their families or which could have been interpreted as disobedience or improper behaviour. No doubt after a number of attempts to get the errant member to toe the line the unfamiliar environment of the British institution and estrangement from the family were resorted to as a means of silencing the challenge of the junior member to the established order of the family. The member was banished but not abandoned as the youngster was valuable to the family, at the very least as a source of productive and/or reproductive labour.

Permanent admissions

> Bhugia. Mania. 40. caste. Service. 15th Jany/63.
> 1863. Sent in by City Magistrate at the request of her husband who is
> a sweeper at the Martinière College. She has been insane for years but
> has recently become wholly unmanageable She roams about picking up
> all sorts of filth and rubs herself over with excrement – at home she is
> entirely intolerable.
> June 1864. This woman is much the same, I see no reasonable hope
> of her ultimate recovery.
> Jany 1870. No better is likely to remain and die an inmate of the
> Asylum.[45]

The idea that admission to the asylum was being used by the Indian community as a disciplinary measure is difficult to sustain for
those cases where the patient is left to die in the institution. Another explanation is needed for those abandoned.

The work of Nancy Waxler, who has studied mental illness in
modern day Sri Lanka, contains a number of insights which offer
an explanation as to why Indians were abandoning members of
their families to the alien institution. She concludes that 'deviance
and the sanctions society uses serve integrating functions in small
societies',[46] going on to state that

> the peasant family that provides treatment for its mentally ill member
> is, at the same time, effectively strengthening its own family structure
> by creating obligations between the patient and family, obligations that
> must be fulfilled later . . . In this sense the family group is further inte-
> grated by the fact of the child's illness.[47]

While a mental illness incident in the family can actually be the
occasion of the group bonding itself as a unit, long-term disorder
tended to have other consequences:

> Both beliefs and practices press the mentally ill person toward return to
> normality . . . In Sri Lanka for example the costs of remaining sick for
> long periods after appropriate treatment are much greater than the costs
> of return to normality; those who do remain chronically ill are threat-
> ened not only with barren lives, but also, ultimately, by lack of food
> and shelter and, most significant, loss of family ties.[48]

While it would obviously be very difficult to compare modern Sri
Lankan villages with mid-nineteenth century North Indian ones,
the model she derives from her study seems to offer an explanation of the patients abandoned to the asylum in the Lucknow case

notes. The case notes from Lucknow of those who are abandoned to the asylum seem to show that they had exhibited long-term disorder. This was the case with Bhugia who was committed by her husband when her behaviour worsened after years of problems and also appears to be the case with Bhoondoo:

> Bhoondoo. Dementia. 35. caste. service. 16 June/63.
> Sent in from Cantonment Joint Magistrate. His mother states he has been getting worse for the last two years, and is now unsafe. Cannot be trusted for one moment alone, and is sometimes violent.
> 20th August. Died of chronic dysentery.[49]

Using these patients then it is possible to suggest that in North India, as in the Sri Lanka of Waxler's study, those suffering with long-term mental disorders were viewed as a burden to be removed permanently from the family. It must be remembered that the minority of such evictions from the family would have been into the asylum. The majority would have been onto the street, which accounts for the number of wandering lunatics for which the British built the asylum in the first place.

It could be then that these are examples of Indians sending those they consider to be mentally ill into the British asylum. But they were not sent in because the Indians had any faith in the Western modes of therapy. They were being sent in not for treatment but for care, in other words there was no expectation of cure on the part of the families when these patients were consigned to the asylum of the British. There was the expectation that the cast off relatives or friends would at least be fed and given a bed, the family no longer being willing to provide for them.

Conclusion

Studies of colonial medical projects in India tend to show that the initial response of the indigenous communities was to reject Western medical interventions. Mark Harrison concluded for example that 'the testimonies of both Europeans and Indians indicate that hostility or indifference towards sanitary regulations persisted in most areas of India',[50] and David Arnold's account of smallpox vaccination projects emphasizes the 'Indian antipathy to vaccination and the coercive, unheeding system of colonialism it was taken to represent'.[51] Both however also show how it was elite Indians whose acceptance of parts of Western medicine ensured that the colonial state was able to negotiate the penetration of its medical projects into Indian society. As such what is left is an image of non-elite Indians resorting to 'riot and resistance' when confronted by Western medicine or else those who did engage with it amongst non-elite groups were characteristically the 'mendicant class and prostitutes',[52] who were hardly representative of local Indian communities as a whole.

These emphases in looking at the responses of Indians to Western medicine are largely the result of the sorts of projects that have been examined. Large-scale interventions like public health projects, vaccination programmes and the measures taken in the face of epidemics involved the sudden reorganization of large populations using coercive measures so it comes as no surprise that reactions to these were often dramatic. However these large-scale interventions were not necessarily typical of colonial medicine as both Arnold and Harrison seem to acknowledge in the few pages that they devote to dispensaries in India. By 1860 Arnold reckons that almost 300 000 people were annually attending the 46 dispensaries in the Madras Presidency[53] and Harrison shows that in 1867 a similar number visited the 61 institutions of Bengal.[54] Yet the reactions and responses of the Indian community to these small-scale and low-priority but nevertheless well attended and much used sites on the interface of colonial medicine and Indian society are summarized in a few lines by both authors. Harrison limits himself to showing how the dispensaries failed to attract female members of the local community. Arnold decides that the factors which lay behind low status Indians using the dispensaries in such numbers was either that they lacked the religious and cultural sensitivities of elite Indians or that they 'became patients less from choice than from desperation or because the police or their European employers sent them there'.[55]

Like the dispensary, the asylum was only one of the responsibilities of the European Civil Surgeon at that station,[56] it was commonly administered on a day to day basis by Indian staff and it was the subject of constant carping by the colonial authorities about its finances and its utility.[57] For the most part it was the subaltern classes of Indians who were dealing with these institutions, 'the three classes whence the largest number are received are ryots, servants and beggars.'[58] In other words this chapter has looked at ordinary Indians interacting with the local, isolated institutions of colonial medicine rather than with its grand projects.

Quite simply, the Indians featured interacting with the asylum were going about their business, the homeless seeking shelter, parents disciplining errant juniors, communities passing on the burden and cost of useless members. In the course of pursuing these mundane and rather unspectacular agendas they were coopting the colonial space, the isolated medical outpost of Empire, into their worlds. There are no new forms of consciousness here, there is no political control or corresponding reactive political action. There is little evidence of the desperation or the state coercion described by Arnold. Various members of Indian society were carrying on their day to day lives and making use of whatever local resources, in this case those supplied by the colonial state, were available for them to get on with those lives. Indeed there is also little evidence that the local communities realized what sort of an institution the lunatic asylum was let alone decided that they would abandon their own understandings of mental illness and appropriate therapy. There is no reason to believe then that Indians were using the asylum for specifically medical reasons. Rather, the Indian community's use of the asylum reflected their willingness to try out all available options when endeavouring to sort out common problems like subsistence and family discipline.

In considering these responses to the low priority local institution, which was in many cases the typical incursion of colonial medicine into local societies and the point at which many indigenous people would have had their only contact with Western medicine, it is difficult to avoid the conclusion that colonial medicine was far from being a force for change. James Paul described the unintended consequences of the introduction of western medicine as the stimulation of new forms of consciousness or political action. This certainly does not seem to be the case in looking at the evidence of Indians admitting Indians into the asylums. Rather the unintended consequence of the introduction of the asylum into Indian communities seems to have been that the institution was itself colonized and reshaped by the routine concerns of local society.

6
Indians inside Asylums: Staff, Patients and Power

He refers in a loud, screaming voice + extra anger to my having once had him put into a bag for restraint. When I smiled he said as much as,
'Now laugh, I will make you cry'.
They say he is never violent except when he sees Europeans, though sometimes he gets angry. He has not been so angry for a very long time. They say he sometimes gets abortive attacks of epilepsy. The Hosp. Asst. has not seen them.[1]

Such episodes, this one taken from the case note for Jeeobadh Koomar who was admitted to the Lucknow asylum in 1869, demonstrate the difficulties and also the possibilities of exploring the responses and reactions of Indians within the asylum. The first point to note is that much of the information that the British medical officer has recorded on the case note about the patient comes from Indians. The 'they' in the case note are the attendants at the asylum who would have been employed from the local population. The fact that it is they who can supply the information on the patient's usual state, that he is 'never violent', and it is they who can point out the exceptions to this rule is significant. This emphasizes that it was Indian personnel rather than the single British doctor who had the day to day contact with the inmates of the institution and who would have been in charge of the routines of the place. The staff is one distinct group whose actions need to be considered in looking at Indians inside the asylums.

The second issue that arises is the question of how to interpret the evidence of what the Indian inmates are supposed to have said and done. Chapter 1 showed how the case notes were constructions of colonial imaginations rather than objective renderings of the real world. Yet to completely ignore Indian voices in these documents, however fragmented and refracted, is to neglect the possibility of exploring subaltern histories at the point of contact with a colonial institution. Ignoring fragments of patients' voices is also unsatisfying for the medical historian, 'a history written only with reference to the activities of physicians is seriously incomplete, as it ignores the experience of the great number of men and women who made up the asylum.'[2] This chapter will explore the Indian actions and voices recorded in the colonial documents to consider whether they reveal anything other than the colonial and medical imagination.

In looking at the evidence of what the inmates said and did it is necessary to deal with the issue of what to do with voices that have been marginalized as 'insane'. In other words the question arises of whether the ramblings of a lunatic or his/her explosions of anger are representative of anything more than the tussles of a disturbed individual with his/her personal demons and delusions. There are three interconnected responses to this.

The first is that any attempt to discount the experiences of those who are mad on the basis that they are lacking in reason or that their responses to the world are non-rational is an endorsement of the much discredited reification as the only proper subject in history of the 'unified and freely choosing individual who is the normative male subject of Western bourgeois liberalism.'[3] Shirley Orter, for example, points out that this subject, 'the freely choosing individual, is an ideological construct, in multiple senses – because the person is culturally (and socially, historically, politically and so forth) constructed; because few people have the power to freely choose very much; and so forth.'[4] To dismiss the experiences of the mad because they were mad is to comply with discourses developed in the nineteenth century in the West which relegated madness to an illness and thereby emptied that state of significance. This was a period described as one when 'compared to the incessant dialogue of reason and madness during the Renaissance . . . silence was absolute; there was no longer any common language between madness and reason.'[5] Such a concern is not necessarily pertinent here though as there is a second response to the idea that the actions and words of those deemed lunatic might not be representative of anything more than private and personalized nightmares. As has already been suggested in Chapters 3 and 5, it is rarely clear that those incarcerated in the institution were indeed mentally ill. The people inside the asylum were there for political and social rather than medical reasons because British doctors, magistrates or jailors, or indeed Indian individuals, elders or husbands, had sought to negotiate behaviour through use of the asylum that was to them deviant (rather than insane) or situations that were threatening to them.

That is why the above case note is so important. It is one of the few which makes explicit the connection between the 'lunatic' classification and the political nature of the behaviour that has led to that classification. As with the designation of an act as 'criminal' so with the designation of an act as 'lunatic,' the label denies the action political significance or meaning. The medicalization of an action empties it of importance as it transforms it into a symptom of a disorder to which the normal individual is being subjected and serves to deny that it is the deliberate and direct statement of opposition of a fully functioning person. Hence, Jeeobadh Koomar's fury and anger at Europeans is neutralized by his being medicalized. Instead of his violence being represented as the forceful expression of anti-colonial antipathy and his threat being a potent statement of rural India's desire to subvert and avenge the colonial relationship it is reproduced on a case note as the utterings of an 'excitable idiot.'[6] If the historian were to disallow the experiences and voices of the Indians who were classified as 'lunatics' simply because the colonial authorities has used that classification then the historian would become implicated in the process where 'colonial power exercised itself in part through its capacity to silence the historical record of the subaltern classes, representing spectacular forms of popular resistance as pathologies.'[7]

A third point that might be raised in connection with the issue of how to interpret the actions and reactions of those deemed lunatic is that those who were truly insane raise interesting questions for discussions of historical agency. Without going into the question of what madness is at length here it would seem that there are certainly those who have organic conditions which result in variations on the standard model of brain structure and which act to influence behaviour.

An example of such an organic condition would be meningoencephalitis of tertiary syphilis[8] or what was called in the nineteenth century 'general paralysis of the insane.' The impact of the disease on the structure of the membranes of the brain has behavioural ramifications:

'Confusion and impairment of memory are common. The patient becomes inefficient, often anxious and nervous and may be thought to be neurotic.'[9]

This behavioural evidence of a physiological state when placed in a social context might easily be interpreted as a reaction to that context. Consider Peloo, a case reported as 'paralysis of the insane' by Dr Wise in the *Indian Medical Gazette* in 1869:

> While under observation at Gowhatty, the civil surgeon reported that he had an incoherent and unsettled manner; that he talked nonsense, that he objected to wear clothes, that he wallowed in the mud, that he was threatening in his behaviour, and very capricious as regards food.[10]

His behaviour in the dispensary could well be seen as resistance to the order of the colonial hospital, as he refused to adopt the dress of the institution, reply in coherent ways and indeed seems to have been positively aggressive on occasions. Yet if this case was correctly diagnosed then Peloo's behaviour was simply a manifestation of a reordering of the structures of his body and his actions had nothing to do with the social context in which he was acting. Indeed, there is every reason to suppose that the diagnosis was indeed accurate as the post-mortem account included by Dr Wise does include observations on the state of the brain which suggest some sort of cereberal transformation: 'The membranes were not coherent. The arachnoid was found distended by a jelly-like effusion, which here and there was of a milky colour.'[11]

An example like that of Peloo is interesting in light of recent discussions of historical agency. These have reached the stage where

> from a theoretical point of view we need a subject who is at once culturally and historically constructed, yet from a political perspective, we would wish this subject to be capable of acting in some sense 'autonomously' not simply in conformity to dominant cultural norms and rules, or within the patterns that power inscribes. But this autonomous actor may not be defined as acting from some hidden well of innate 'will' or consciousness that has somehow escaped cultural shaping and ordering. In fact, such an actor is not only possible but 'normal' for the simple reason that neither 'culture' itself nor the regimes of power that are imbricated in cultural logics and experiences can ever be wholly consistent or totally determining ... every actor always carries around enough disparate and contradictory strands of knowledge and passion so as always to be in a potentially critical position. Thus the practices of everyday life may be seen as replete with petty rebellions and inchoate discontent.[12]

While a difference between the 'passion' that is identified by the authors as an important factor in the disruption of the cultural and historical determinants and the 'will' that transcends and must therefore not be mentioned is not made at all clear the above statement could be read as wishful thinking or indeed an attempt by linguistic sleight of hand to reintroduce the transcendent 'will.' However, it might be suggested that novel mental states caused by physiological factors could account for the actions and attitudes of individual agents which serve to disrupt and distort the cultural and historical structures. In other words, the 'passion' of individuals which results in them acting as agents to creatively interact with the environment of their communities and lifestyles can be accounted for without reference to an innate and essential human 'will'. A study of those in whom the organic factor in behaviour and mental functioning is most evident demonstrates that there may well be other factors behind human actions and perceptions than cultural and historical circumstances.

Overall then, there are a variety of reasons to explore the experiences and responses of those Indians inside the asylum and this chapter. These explorations will first look at the Indian workers in the colonial institution and will then focus on the responses of those Indians incarcerated by the British authorities.

The asylum staff

It has been suggested that it is the attendants and wardens that lived within the asylums who hold the key to understanding asylum experiences rather than the professional medical men who were given the charge of the institutions but rarely visited or chose to organize from a distance. In an important article Richard Russell points out that in Britain

> the nursing staff were indeed the backbone of the asylum ... for a brief time during the latter part of the nineteenth century it seems reasonable to suppose that the nursing staff were the most vital part of the whole asylum business.[13]

Indeed he goes on to conclude that 'it may be that the asylum system upon which the whole lunacy profession rested ... was being slowly transformed by new ideas brought from below, by the nursing staff, whose origins and attitudes the men at the top were not fully able to control.'[14]

This idea, that the subordinate staff had considerable power in the day-to-day routine of asylum administration which may have served to transform in practice the regimes and schemes devised in isolation by the medical profession is especially interesting in the colonial context where the subordinate staff would have consisted largely of members of the colonized population. Yet this is a relatively undeveloped theme both in the work on asylums in the colonial context and indeed in studies of medical administration in the colonial context as a whole. Harriet Deacon does mention the staff at the asylum on Robben Island but only in the context of a pay dispute amongst European subordinates.[15] Waltraud Ernst concedes that in India 'only in "native lunatic asylums" were Indian assistants customarily entrusted with the day-to-day care of Indian and lower-class Eurasian patients.'[16] However she does not explore the implications of this situation. David Arnold mentions an interesting incident where 'the most menial servants of Western medicine,'[17] the Doms who worked in the dissecting rooms of the College Hospital in Calcutta, resisted the attempts of the British to conduct a post-mortem on one of their own number. However, he uses this as a pretext to explore Indian society's reactions to Western medicine as a whole rather than to examine the impact on medical institutions of such resistance by subordinate medical staff to the designs of doctors.

The most comprehensive attempt to explore the experiences of members of the colonized population who acted as medical subordinates is a study done by Maryinez Lyons of African auxiliaries in East Africa. Lyons shows how the intentions of the European authorities in instituting medical programmes and facilities were often frustrated by the auxiliaries who were sent out to administer them. These Africans had their own agendas which they pursued using the power and the resources available to them as representatives of state medicine, 'the biomedical technology was especially attractive to individuals who wished for status and influence.'[18] The pursuit of these agendas would have resulted in preferential access to treatment for favoured social groups, the development of a market in pilfered medical supplies and so on. Quite simply, the objectives of the Africans sent out to implement colonial medical projects did not always coincide with those of the Europeans who had planned the medical projects. These independent agendas often had the result that colonial medical schemes became distorted or were even thwarted.

It is clear that by 1880 the Indian staff of asylums were considerable bodies of people. At the largest of the asylums at Dullunda near Calcutta the staff under the British medical officer was as follows:

 1 Deputy Superintendent
 1 Matron
 1 Writer
 1 Native Doctor
 1 Compounder
 5 Jemadars
24 Keepers
 2 Hospital keepers
 4 Durwans
 1 Hukara
 1 Lamplighter
 1 Mallies
 3 Cooks
 1 Baker
 1 Washerman
12 Mahters
 6 Mehteranis
 2 Barbers
 3 Bhistees[19]

In the year 1880 this staff had to attend to a daily average of about 215 patients. Even in the smaller institutions the staff were fairly numerous. At Delhi in 1880 there were 73 patients in the asylum at the end of the year and the staff were listed as:

1 Deputy Super
1 Native Doctor
1 Head Warder
2 1st Class Warders
3 2nd Class Warders
3 3rd Class Warders
3 4th Class Warders
1 Cook
1 Assistant-Cook
1 Gardener
1 Bhisti
1 Dhobi
2 Sweepers
1 Barber
1 Matron
2 Assistant Matrons[20]

The staff in the smaller institution numbered 25 then and like the larger institution the patient to staff ratio was about 3:1. It is therefore not difficult to see then how the day to day running of the institution was almost entirely in the hands of Indians. Indeed, only in the instance of the asylum at Madras does a European medical officer appear to have had the asylum as his sole responsibility in this period so it was only there that the asylum would have had the constant presence of a British medical officer. It was the norm that the local Civil Surgeon should have the charge of the asylum as just one of his many duties. The time and attention that the asylum received from such an officer is likely, through sheer pressure of work, to have been minimal. J. Howard Thornton, who was a Civil Surgeon in India in the 1870s, wrote in his memoirs of the tasks that the medical officer of the station was expected to attend to:

> The day after my arrival I took over my duties which included the management of the district jail, containing more than four hundred prisoners, as well as the superintendence of the Arrah dispensary, and several branch dispensaries in different parts of the district, the medical charge of the district police and other civil establishments and a fair amount of private practice in the station and neighbourhood ... In addition to the various duties pertaining to the office of Civil Surgeon ... I was one of the municipal commissioners of the town of Arrah ... I was also a member of the district school committee ... I was ex-officio, police surgeon, and all examinations of police cases as well as post mortem examinations had to be performed by me ... quarrels and fights about boundaries, water, straying cattle, grazing rights, and many other disputed matters were so common in that part of India that nearly every day I had to examine persons who had been injured in these conflicts ... All these cases involved my subsequent attendance in the different courts of justice for the purpose of giving medical evidence.
>
> It will thus be seen that the time of a Civil Surgeon in India is pretty well occupied even in an ordinary station like Arrah. In a large station like Patna, where the Civil Surgeon has in addition a lunatic asylum under his charge, and a medical school to superintend the work is much heavier and some of it must necessarily be left in the hands of subordinates.[21]

Sometimes one of these subordinates at the asylum would have been a European in the capacity as Deputy Superintendent or Overseer, and the reports for Patna throughout the 1870s suggest that such a number sometimes doubled: 'Mr Nowlan as Overseer and Mrs Nowlan as Matron worked steadily and faithfully throughout the year, and I have much pleasure in commending them to the Surgeon General.'[22] In these cases there would have been a constant European presence at the asylum, albeit a small one. However, the same report from

Bengal in which that statement was made also includes the following remarks about the asylum at Berhampore: 'The Overseer, Baboo Mohendro Nath Roy, regarding whose character and fitness for the post he occupies I have fully expressed in former reports, continues to perform his duties in an efficient and honest manner.'[23] It would seem then that even the most senior of the staff who were permanently at the asylum could sometimes be Indian.

The composition of the Indian staff seems to have been rather mixed. There are hints that some of the Native Doctors were formerly attached to military units: '1st Class Hospital Assistant Lutchman Singh still maintains the high opinion I found regarding him on the occasion of previous reports, and he has seen much service and was in the Bailey Guard during the Mutiny',[24] reported Dr Cannon at Lucknow in 1872. Similarly at the asylum in Dullunda Dr Payne noted that 'the native doctor of whom I had reported unfavourably was moved during the year and his place supplied by Sheikh Bahadoor, a man who bore a high character in the military service.'[25] Indeed the military connection was also evident in the making up of the subordinate staff:

> The conduct of the native establishment has been excellent. Slowly progressive change has taken place under the present scale of wages in the class of men who take the service. Some of the new men had served in various capacities under the overseer in the horse artillery in former years. A few are Punjabees who have taken their discharge from regiments quartered in this neighbourhood and being contented with the service have summoned others from long distances. The general result is that a staff of servants very different from, and in every respect greatly superior to, that of former days is in course of formation.[26]

In a similar vein the staff at Hazaribagh seem to have seen service elsewhere in the British system. This came to light in a report where the superintendent 'expresses the obligation he is under to Mr Parry Davis, District Superintendent of Police, who procured jemadars for him (three of whom were police head constables of superior character) and arranged a comprehensive system of discipline as to reliefs etc.'[27]

However, it was not the case that the asylum staff was invariably drawn from ex-servicemen. Dr Fairweather at the Delhi asylum bemoaned the fact that 'there is not much to be said about the barkandazes and keepers, who, from the smallness of their pay, are generally men who have failed to get employment elsewhere.'[28] Likewise, the Inspector-General of Prisons in Burma whose responsibility it was to staff the asylum at Rangoon was disdainful of the class that the pay on offer would attract. However, it appears that he had devised a way of getting around this:

> As will be noticed, I have introduced a large convict element into the constitution of the establishment; and I have done so, because in the first place, I consider that by this measure the Chief Commissioner's instructions to observe the strictest economy in framing my estimates may be closely adhered to; and in the second, because the Asylum will in this way obtain in its minor offices the services of men much more trustworthy, much more intelligent, and much more orderly than any whom it is possible to find amongst the class of free natives of India which alone would be disposed to take service in the institution.[29]

Whatever the exact constitution of the Indian staff in the various asylums however, it is clear that Indians made up the bulk of the staff in all the asylums who routinely dealt with the inmate population. Indeed, many held positions of seniority and responsibility within those institutions. As such Indians were in a position to frustrate the plans of the medical officers for the patients and it seems that they did indeed resist and subvert colonial agendas. They did this in two interconnected ways, by refusing to meet the basic demands of work discipline expected by the British and by actively disrupting the treatment regimes devised by the colonial authorities.

The basic demands of colonial work discipline or what has been called the 'norm of [the] conscientious worker,'[30] seem to have been often ignored by the asylum staff who were reluctant to give their all for so little reward. Some instances of this seemed fairly innocuous even to the British superintendent, Dr Birch for example reporting that 'the keepers and other subordinates, on the whole, worked well. Sleeping while on watch at night is their chief offence.'[31] The attendants at Patna seem to have incurred the displeasure of the superintendent there with some regularity. In 1878 for example the end of year report noted that 'three jemadars, eleven keepers and two mehters were fined for petty offences, one jemadar resigned, one washerwoman and one carpenter were dismissed for neglect of duty.'[32] The medical officer at the Delhi institution gave an account of his staff in 1875 which shows how Indian personnel consistently resisted attempts to impose on them schedules and duties which did not suit them:

The barkandazes and keepers are indolent and troublesome. I cannot get them to be careful with or vigilant over the patients. They are repeatedly being fined for staying away without leave beyond hours, for neglect, untidiness and remissness in guarding and tending the lunatics.[33]

Neither was resistance to the work discipline expected by the British medical officers in the asylum restricted to those Indians working in the menial positions in the institutions. The superintendent at the Dullunda asylum wrote in 1870:

The native doctor of whom I had reported unfavourably was moved during the year and his place supplied by Sheikh Bahadoor, a man who bore a high character in the military service, and I have no doubt deserved it; but the hospital system of a regiment does not create the habits that are required in the asylum. There cases of illness are brought to the hospital or to the notice of the subordinate, whose business it is to attend only where his attention is called for. Here he is mainly useful in spontaneously searching for illness among the inhabitants of the place, without which search it often progresses unknown. To keep up an unremitting search for illness throughout the day is a practice which does not commend itself to the understanding or the inclination of a man who is accustomed to consider his day's work done, or nearly so, when the surgeon's visit is over. [34]

The hint of frustration in the passage would seem to suggest that Sheikh Bahadoor was withstanding the efforts of the superintendent to transform his working habits from that of waiting in the infirmary for new cases to arrive to that of active surveillance of the institution's population. Similarly in 1871 the report for the asylums in Bengal for the previous year concentrated on the comments of the superintendent at Dacca:

The native doctor, Sheikh Abdoollah, whose conduct is unfavourably commented on, has been removed, and a more promising young man appointed. On the subject of native doctors for lunatic asylums, Mr Buckle remarks as follows in his covering memorandum: 'The fact is, that a higher amount of intelligence, and a more careful performance of their duty, is required both from the native doctor and the attendants at a lunatic asylum than in any other situation. It is almost impossible to make the native doctor understand that it is his business to be constantly watching the insane, to notice who is sick, who more dull and depressed than usual, and that his duty lies far beyond waiting at the hospital until the sick are brought to him. I certainly think that the pay of the native doctor is too low to secure or retain a good man. The duties here are far more difficult and responsible than those in a jail hospital, where the pay is the same – Rs.25. I think the at least Rs.40 should be the salary of asylum native doctor where the number of inmates exceeds 100.'[35]

Again then there is the sense that even the senior members of staff at the asylums were capable of ignoring British attempts to get them to take on more work for much the same money.

Naturally any refusal by the Indian staff in the asylums to take on work or to perform the tasks that the British expected of them in the asylum would have had implications for the efficacy of the treatment regimes that were discussed in the Chapter 4. Indeed there is plenty of evidence that these treatment regimes were actively subverted by the Indian staff.

There were various means by which the British made the asylum staff aware of what they were supposed to be doing so that any failure by the staff to perform certain tasks can be seen as conscious refusal rather than unwitting non-compliance. As has already been suggested in the above extracts there was a fine system operating in many asylums where failures to perform the expected duty were penalized. In this way Indian staff would have learnt what was expected from those of whom an example had been made. More positive attempts were made however to school the staff in what they were being employed to do. For example as early as 1856 a superintendent had set out a clear set of instructions for the asylum staff and the means by which they would be made aware of these instructions, even if they were illiterate:

Rules for the Guidance of the Subordinate Establishment of the Asylum at Dullunda.

i. The European Overseer, the Native Doctor, and Servants male and female, are strictly enjoined invariably to treat the patients with the greatest kindness; to abstain from harsh language, threats, abuse, all acts of oppression, blows or any other acts. They are to remember that the unfortunate patients are of unsound mind and not responsible agents.
ii. When the conduct of a Patient becomes violent and dangerous to himself and others, the Hospital Servants will, in the absence of the Super, report the circs to the Overseer who will immediately visit the patient. Should the Overseer consider restraint to be absolutely necessary for the safety of the Patient himself or others, temporary seclusion may accordingly be applied. But in such case, the Overseer will report the circumstance to the Superintendent.
iii. Clubs, sticks, weapons, sharp edged or pointed tools are strictly prohibited from being introduced into the Asylum.
iv. Such patients as may be permitted to assist in the kitchen and garden are not to be trusted with knives or tools with which they may commit injury.
v. Visitors to the Patients are to be admitted with the permission of the Magistrate of the 24 Pergunnahs or of the Superintendent.
vi. All complaints relating to the Patients or to the Hospital Servants

are immediately to be brought to the notice of the Overseer, who will take the earliest opportunity to report to the Superintendent.

vii. The overseer will see that the preceding rules are strictly observed and a copy in English and in Bengallee is to be kept suspended in the office. The native Doctor will at the monthly Muster read to the Hospital Establishment a Bengallee translation of the preceding rules.

signed, T. Cantor and H.D.H. Fergusson, Fort William Jan 1 1856.[36]

Instructions seem to have been issued elsewhere, the superintendent at Bareilly stating that 'I need hardly say that no violence on the part of the attendants is ever allowed, and they understand that a blow, or indeed any kind of harshness or rough usage is visited by immediate dismissal.'[37] Some asylums seem to have gone further than simply issue a series of orders and devised ways of skilling their staff. For example, the Surgeon General in Madras noted in 1874 that, from the asylum at Vizagapatam, 'a Head Warder, with one female and two male warders, were sent for special training in the Madras Institution.'[38]

There is evidence then that the Indian staff at the asylums received at the very least instructions as to what to do in the asylum if not actual training in how to go about their jobs. There is also plenty of evidence however that the staff often did not create on the ground the asylum environment that the British medical officers described in their reports as desirable.

In an annual report for the asylum at Waltair the superintendent pointed out that the

> conduct of warders and servants has been upon the whole fair, with three exceptions, a male warder, female warder and female cooly who were dismissed and prosecuted for striking patients. I hope these dismissals and prosecutions – in each case a conviction was obtained – will act as a deterrent against the commission of such offence in future.[39]

Similarly at Benares the superintendent had to report in 1867 that 'one of the two Jemadars was dismissed some months ago for striking a patient',[40] and at Dacca 'the keeper who struck a lunatic in the face with his fist was reported to the police, and a local enquiry was made, but the case went no further for want of legal evidence. He was nevertheless dismissed.'[41] Perhaps most illustrative of all was the case brought up by Dr Payne at Dullunda, the asylum where the system of reading out the rules to the staff had begun in the 1850s:

> For the first time during an incumbency of ten years I am compelled to
> report a death from violence. A maniac was brutally ill treated by a
> peon, and died from the effects of it. The peon was convicted and im-
> prisoned and thus was obtained the only possible satisfaction which
> can follow the occurrence of such a case.[42]

It was demonstrated in Chapter 4 that the British intended to
base the asylum regime in India on firm but kind treatment in
keeping with contemporary views on the management of the insane in Europe. Indian staff showed themselves more than capable
of frustrating those designs and disrupting that regime. Indeed, other
elements of the British plans for the treatment of the inmates were
resisted by the attendants. Putting the inmates to work was an
important component in the ideal system. The superintendent at
Delhi had to write a report in 1876 which suggested that it had
been difficult to get the staff there to cooperate with him in setting
up projects for the incarcerated:

> In the treatment of the insane the chief reliance has been put upon
> healthy occupation and amusement. After a long struggle, and with every
> kind of opposition thrown in the way by the Asylum establishment, I at
> last succeeded in starting some manufactures in July last.[43]

The agendas, even survival strategies, of Indian attendants is most
obvious in the frustration of a further element of the asylum regime which had as its focus the body of the inmate. The medical
officers thought that attention to diet in order to establish physical
health in the patient was central to a successful asylum. The superintendent at Delhi stated in 1870 that 'the diet has been liberal.
Good, well ground wheaten flour chappaties, fit for any breakfast,
four each – three in the morning and one in the evening – together with dall and vegetables four times a week, and a stew of
meat and vegetables three times a week.'[44] He pointed out again in
1872 that 'good feeding, great kindness and indulgence of every
harmless kind'[45] were the central tenets of his institution.

The statement in the report of 1875 comes as some surprise
then:

> I regret I cannot report favourably about the subordinate establishment.
> The assistant matron, the cook and a keeper have been discharged for
> stealing the lunatics food and several of the burkundazes and keepers
> have been fined or dismissed for carelessness or harsh treatment of the
> lunatics under their charge.[46]

In other words certain of the staff had taken the opportunity that access to the supplies of the asylum gave them to supplement poor incomes with acquired perks. This opportunism was not restricted to the staff in Delhi either. Surgeon-Major Birch at Hazaribagh in Bengal complained in 1878 that 'two cooks have been summarily dismissed for this offence and another was prosecuted, but that pilfering still goes on I fear is the case, notwithstanding the measures taken to prevent it. Only a few days ago the Overseer detected two of the cooks stealing the meat which ought to have been issued to the patients.'[47]

While such theft can be linked to the survival strategies of the subordinate staff this last example hints at other reasons for them to be removing certain items of the patient's diet. While superintendents may have been extolling the virtues of 'a stew of meat and vegetables three times a week' few others in the asylum would have shared his enthusiasm for cooked flesh. Most Indians would have been committed to a vegetarian diet for cultural and religious reasons in this period and as was suggested in Chapter 4 the British medical officer may have been simply ignorant of this or indeed could have had ulterior motives for insisting on including meat in the inmate's meals. The possibility is raised, in the above example at least where it is specifically the meat which is being removed by the cooks, that the Indian staff were acting for the benefit of the inmates. The attendants knew that a refusal to eat what was presented to them could often result in punishment or forced feeding for the inmates.[48] It could be that the staff were acting out of sympathy for the patients by removing the offending flesh before it was presented to them as their dinner.

Whatever the explanation in this example, it seems certain that the bodily treatment of the asylum regime was often disrupted by those members of the establishment who were supposed to administer it. Indeed as the set of extracts quoted from Delhi shows, the statements of the superintendent in the reports about the systems operating within the asylum were sometimes simply rhetoric. The decisions of the Indian staff, who often had their own ideas about what should go on, actually determined conditions and experiences on the ground. While the reports of the superintendent claimed that 'good feeding' and 'great kindness' were the basis of the preferred asylum regime it appears from those reports that the staff were actually removing the food and sometimes dealing severely with the patients. In other words they were subverting the designs and objectives of the regime in the asylums because of their own agendas and through the power that they had as those charged with the day to day running of the institutions.

It must be remembered that this power to shape events within the asylum was not always used by Indians to resist the designs of the British. Often the response of the staff seems to have been to work hard to make the regime tick over and to make sure that the asylum ran smoothly. While certain of the 'native doctors' mentioned above seem unwilling to take on the additional tasks connected with serving in an asylum there were those who were happy to muck in. Surgeon Major Shircore reported:

> Native Doctor Rutoo is well spoken of, having been attached to the Moydapore dispensary for 29 years, and has been attached to the Berhampore Asylum since its opening in 1874. He is well acquainted with all the details of duty, and his willingness to help in the general management of the lunatics renders him a useful officer.[49]

The civil as opposed to the medical staff could also show considerable accomplishment in their roles, the superintendent at Cuttack being happy to note that 'the conduct of the establishment during the year has been uniformly good. The darogah has been in charge for the past 15 years and has performed his duties to my entire satisfaction; he possesses remarkable tact in managing the insanes and in keeping the minor establishment up to their work.'[50] In his report for the same year the superintendent at Dullunda insisted on including the following note:

> The head clerk, Oparva Narain Bhattacharjee has been indefatigable throughout the year, giving in time of need much more time and labor to the asylum than can be legitimately demanded of him, and never complaining however heavy the additional calls have been or however irregular his hours of rest.[51]

Some staff were considered indispensable because of their personal qualities. In 1870 the Deputy Inspector-General of Hospitals in Lucknow wrote that 'Dr Cannon reports very favorably of 1st class Native Doctor Luchman Sing; but he is bent with age and disease and I only refrain from invaliding him on account of Dr Cannon's assurances as to his efficiency and usefulness, and knowledge of the working of the institution.'[52] It was explained in 1874 by Dr Cannon, by then the Deputy Surgeon-General of the Lucknow Circle that the conduct and qualifications of First Class Hospital Assistant Luchman Singh have always been reported well of by every medical officer under whom he has served, and I quite endorse the opinion of Dr Ray that although old and a sufferer from chronic rheumatism, he is admirably qualified for managing insanes both from his superior tact and good temper, and on this account his services are more valuable in an Asylum than those of a younger and less experienced man.[53]

It seems that often Indians were willing to take on the extra work associated with employment in the asylum, to devote extra hours to their duties where necessary and to ignore the debilities of age and infirmity in order to get on with their jobs at the asylum.

There are obviously difficulties in dealing with this sort of evidence and in deciding what was going on in the asylums. The accounts of the medical officers could be dismissed as self-serving and written to give impressions of competence, so that commendation of subordinates might be exaggerated or individual attendants might be given the blame in order to show the superintendent in a better light. There is no doubt an element of this in the reports, although there was a system of Visitors where local civil and medical officers would inspect institutions like the asylum which would have made consistent subterfuge by the superintendents more difficult. Indeed there are instances where the management of institutions was called into question. So for example, the dietary scale in the Dullunda asylum became a matter of some controversy in 1869 after the Inspector-General of Hospitals in the Lower Provinces of Bengal complained that 'I noticed also that very many of the insanes are exceedingly anaemic and cachetic and there is no doubt in my mind . . . that the system of dieting carried on for a long time in this asylum was a thoroughly inadequate one in relation to the amount of actual labor performed.'[54]

What cannot be doubted is the fact that Civil Surgeons had many other calls on their time in the station and that for larger parts of the day, if not the week, the asylum was in the hands of Indian subordinates and the inmate population was subject to their supervision rather than the direct control of any colonial officer. To underline this it is worth mentioning that the rules for the Lucknow asylum, at which Luchman Singh held sway despite his rheumatism, demanded only that 'the superintendent shall regularly visit the Asylum at least three days in each week.'[55] In these circumstances the Indian staff would have had considerable scope for making decisions and pursuing agendas independent of those sanctioned by the British officers. Significantly the decisions they made and the agendas they pursued often appear to have undermined the avowed intentions of the asylum regime despite evidence that the Indian staff had indeed been made aware of those avowed intentions. It is not difficult to see these as examples of Indians resisting the colonisers' power to impose order even within their own institutions.

However, just as significant is the fact that many Indians worked in the institutions to the satisfaction of the British, satisfaction that appears to be justified where it appears that the results can be measured in material terms. The sale of articles produced at the Dullunda asylum reaped Rs 7205[56] for the asylum in 1880 with an average daily population of 215. This is an extreme example of a system that was operating throughout the asylums of India by the end of the 1870s where even the smaller institutions proved themselves sufficiently organized to produce goods worth over Rs 1000 per annum.[57] The design of such operations might be attributed to the British medical officer but the routine administration of them cannot when it is recalled that he had so much else to do. This administration would have devolved on the subordinate staff who were in the asylum on a daily basis and would have been, with the occasional exception of a European overseer, completely drawn from the Indian community. Superintendents acknowledged as much in their reports, Major Scriven at Lahore making a point of thanking his staff on the occasion of his return to Britain and emphasizing that 'not less to be commended are the jemadar, the compounder and the jamadarni. The jemadar, Mirza Hassam Ali, has been here 13 years. He thoroughly understands the work of the institution and we should have had great difficulty in carrying on the work without him.'[58]

It must not be assumed however that these Indians were any different from those who chose to resist British orders and instructions. They were making the British system work for their own reasons and in pursuit of their own agendas. Sometimes these are obvious, as there are pecuniary rewards on offer for diligence: 'All the servants of the Asylum are at present good and respectable men, and understand their duties thoroughly. They are very badly paid . . . so to encourage them I give them an extra rupee or two per month from the profit fund of the Asylum. I find this plan answers very well.'[59]

Sometimes though, the reasons that Indians had for making the British systems work in the asylums can only be speculated at. The status that a position in the colonial service or access to Western knowledge gave was part of the attraction that persuaded Africans to train as auxiliaries in Lyons's account of the medical services in Uganda and the Belgian Congo.[60] Maybe such a factor influenced Luchman Singh's decision to work on into his old age, as the power of controlling a staff might have been difficult to relinquish or quite simply retirement could have been difficult to contemplate.

Whichever is the case, it is clear that the day-to-day running of the asylums was in the hands of predominantly Indian staff. It is also clear that the Indian attendant could and did resist British attempts to circumscribe his conduct by the issuing of instructions and the threat of dismissal. The result of this would have been that the experience of the inmates of the institution was frequently determined by the agendas and decisions of Indian personnel rather than colonial directives.

Indian patients

> Although many insane persons on first admission yield themselves at once to the order and discipline of the place by the mere force of example and the imitative faculty, which is unimpaired, and take up without difficulty some one of the employments before them, there are others for whom occupation is no less necessary, who require the constant efforts of attendants to keep them at their work and who frequently offer both active and passive resistance.[61]

The patient population also provides interesting examples of resistance to colonial strategies and objectives. These instances of resistance came in three forms, the verbal, the violent and the escape.

As already stated, examples of Indians speaking in colonial documents are obviously problematic, as the methods by which their statements came to be translated, selected and recorded are rarely transparent. However, as was shown with the example of Jeeobadh Koomar which was the focus of the beginning of this discussion of Indian responses, the Indian voice can still raise interesting possibilities even where it is refracted through a colonial text. His case note recorded the moment when he threatened the medical officer who had ordered him restrained in a bag. Even if the medical officer had pared down the context or the content of the entire episode there is still a record of an important moment when the colonial medical officer's authority was contested.

The same might be said of the following passage which appeared in the annual report on the asylums in Bombay in 1874. In a general discussion on the merits of a system of labour in the management of insanes, the superintendent asserts that, 'to us the best sign of improvement is the willingness to work.'[62] He then mentions 'one Seedee, whose hopes of recovery are but small, wants to know if we take him for a coolee when we ask him to work; this man talks for hours to imaginary people.' In this example the patient is denied even a transcription of a translation of his voice and instead his statement is summarized by the superintendent and sandwiched in between two unequivocal confirmations of the man's irrational state. These confirmations offered by the medical officer are designed to silence and discredit the moment of resistance as manifestation of an illness rather than as conscious defiance. Nevertheless, the moment of resistance is still present in the document and is vitally important as it confirms that patients did actively resist the British agenda of putting them to work.

Where inmates would not work this was usually represented as being beyond their control. 'Lunatics with the delusion of greatness strongly impressed on the mind are most difficult to induce to work',[63] insisted Dr Simpson at Dacca thereby assigning their refusal to work to a special kind of lunacy. The case note for Rajoowa at Lucknow represents his unwillingness to work as an inability: 'He was always quiet, never turbulent, but could not be persuaded to do any work – sometimes tried but had no *jee* [sic] for anything.'[64] Even where the inmate was seen to be actively resisting work this was assigned to a failing rather than active reluctance. So for example, Ajjoddhia's case note states that he 'occasionally can be induced to work, refuses apparently from laziness only.'[65] By referring to 'laziness' here Ajjodhia's resistance to work is being linked with a series of racial discourses on the 'lazy native.'[66] which was developed in the colonial encounter. Such a discourse served to represent the refusal of the peoples that the Europeans encountered to fit in with their economic projects as evidence of racial weakness rather than overt resistance.

However Seedee's sense of indignation at being requested to work at some menial task, an indignation which comes through even in a colonial medical document, suggests that patients did actively resist the labour regime of the asylums. Seedee refused to work as he saw it as beneath him and his sardonic reply implies that he was making sure that those who expected him to work knew that he was not malingering or incapacitated. In other words, he was not simply resisting the treatment strategies of the institution, he was making sure that those who expected him to work knew that he was resisting them.

A similar example is that of Hyder Cooly which was reported by the superintendent of the Dullunda asylum:

> Some of them are very interesting from their humour and other pecu-
> liarities. One of these, well known to every visitor of the Asylum, is
> Hyder Cooly; this man has been for some years a cook to the European
> soldiers at Dinapore, where he acquired a vocabulary of about eighty or
> a hundred English words. On the occasion of any European visiting the
> Asylum, Hyder always addresses them in the most absurd jargon of bro-
> ken English that can be imagined, his countenance lighting up by degrees
> to a broad grin. Looking the person he is addressing full in the face he
> generally ends a long rigmarole of incoherent talk with 'go to hell you
> black fellow' and then bursts into a loud laugh. But Hyder is not always
> in a comic vein; at times (but rarely) he is low and melancholy, and in
> tears; he does not then speak in English, but his lugubrious, odd expres-
> sion is almost as ludicrous as when he is in a more happy mood.[67]

A reading which ignores the author's attempts to discredit Hyder Cooly provides a fine example of an Indian happily berating Europeans from the protected status as a 'lunatic.' Only the previous year for example, the same superintendent who wrote the above account had written: 'Civilly incapable and criminally irresponsible the pauper lunatic in custody is exempt from retributive justice and for him sympathy disarms the law.'[68] Safe in this knowledge, Hyder Cooly launched into his diatribe using as much English as he knew, of which some would have been 'absurd' to the asylum Visitors who as officers might not have been familiar with many of the English words he had picked up from the infantrymen. Whether or not he was verbally comprehensible he knew that by drawing himself up to his full physical extent, eyeing the British officer full in the face and issuing the order 'go to hell you black fellow' he had a great way of insulting and berating those from the same class that had insulted and berated him. With a finale that turned the power relations that he had suffered throughout his life on their heads and which ended with a forceful curse, no wonder he allowed himself a loud laugh.

Hyder Cooly's well practised performance is a spectacular example of a low status Indian joyfully avenging the insults of a lifetime by using his special status as a lunatic to abuse the local brass whenever he gets the opportunity. To simply say that it is nothing of the kind because the man is 'mad' is to comply with the project of the superintendent at Dullunda. Although tempted to pass on the vignette the officer still feels it necessary to emphasize, even in a report about lunatics, that the man in question was undoubtedly unstable and therefore not to be taken at face value and this explains the sentence after the punchline which seeks to discredit Hyder as 'odd' and 'ludicrous.' The way that the narrative is constructed provides another good example of the process described above, where resistance is emptied of political meaning by representing it as pathology.

However difficult it is to interpret the voices of Indians which are embedded in sources exclusively authored by colonial officers, it is important not to ignore those fragments. Even where the documents seek to hide the meanings of Indian statements under layers of appropriation, translation and meaning, it is still possible to find instances where Indians verbally resisted the objectives and indeed the relationships of colonialism. A far more active way of resisting the objectives of the asylum though was to simply absent oneself from the institution altogether. Escape seems to have been a fairly common occurrence in some asylums. In 1877 the annual report for the Central Provinces noted that at the Nagpur asylum 'two males discharged themselves by escape, and have not subsequently been captured.'[69] It also mentioned that there had been one escape from the Jubbulpore institution, the other asylum in the administration. In 1878 there was a further escape from Nagpur, but none from Jubbulpore, in 1879 another from Nagpur and two from Jubbulpore and in 1880 Nagpur managed to keep its inmate population intact while Jubbulpore lost three who opted to 'discharge themselves by escape.'

Similarly in Madras there was a tendency for some inmates to opt for a voluntary early release:

> There have been four escapes, of whom only one was recaptured; all were harmless, quiet lunatics, and therefore evaded the vigilance of the warders, whose attention is more specifically directed to the troublesome and dangerous patients. No criminals effected their escape. To obviate the wandering away of the inmates, the aloe fence surrounding the asylum is being repaired and the trench deepened as the cost of a wall, which would alone effectually prevent escapes, is found too heavy.[70]

The superintendent's hopes for the repairs to the hedge and the trench were however dashed in the next twelve months. Indeed his faith in a wall also seems to have been questionable:

There have been five escapes during the year, three of whom were brought back, and of the remaining two, who were admitted as criminals, one was transferred to the ordinary list as his time of imprisonment had expired. These two patients made their escape by getting upon the roof of the latrine, and thence on to the main wall, from which it is supposed they let themselves down by cloths they had borrowed or stolen from other patients. Nothing has since been heard of them although the matter was at once reported to the Police authorities.[71]

Escapees sometimes opted not to give the asylum a chance to work on them and sought their escape without delay, the superintendent at Colaba reporting at one point that 'one lunatic escaped through the ventilator in the roof of his small room three days after his admission into the asylum, and has not yet been captured.'[72] Others decided to make a break for it despite being considered something of an asylum fixture: 'A Gond, named Lalu from Chanda, escaped, though an old inmate of the asylum, and had always been considered harmless and quiet.'[73]

That those who were escaping were not simply wandering off in a daze, but were actively attempting to resist incarceration in the institution is emphasized in the details in instances like the following:

> Moula Buy. Amentia. Servant. Mussul. 27. 7th Jan.
>
> 1861 Jany. A sepoy of the Meerut Regt. – imprisoned for some regimental breach of discipline, was some days in the Jail of Lucknow before transferred him to the asylum – is a slight, tall man of good address + very intelligent. Talks very incoherently + fancies that there was some combination against him.
>
> Feb 13th. Made his escape – apparently with the connivance of his wife – during the night + was some days afterwards brought back from Cawnpore whither he said he had gone to take the air + bathe in the Ganges but that he had suffered so much distress on the road that he would not repeat his walk for some time – is very restless + unsettled. Is no longer a prisoner.
>
> April 13th. In consequence of his continued attempts to escape – he was chained in his ward at night – notwithstanding this + a burkundaz on duty – this morning he was found to have again escaped. A rope ladder, evidently let down by some accomplice, was found suspended from the roof. he had escaped under the projecting eaves + dropped down outside. Has not been retaken. Absconded.[74]

This former soldier was obviously determined not to be locked up by the British authorities and despite recapture and the considerable obstacles presented by the asylum to his attempts to escape it appears that he finally managed it and successfully evaded recapture. Indeed, what is most significant about this example is that there appear to be members of the Indian community outside of the walls involved in facilitating his breakout. It seems then that the flight of individuals from the asylum can in certain cases be seen not just as examples where inmates resisted the colonial decision about their fate. They might also be seen as instances where Indian families and community members resisted those decisions.

An inmate of the Jubbulpore asylum who was mentioned in the end of year report of 1880 seemed similarly determined to resist the British authorities:

> The criminal Mahso as a boy was confined in the Nagpur Jail reformatory wards for murder of a child in the Raipur District; whilst in jail he murdered another juvenile prisoner by driving the end of a pickaxe into the boy's back. For this second murder he was tried and acquitted on the ground of insanity in July 1876. During the whole time that he has been under observation in the asylum he has shown no signs of insanity beyond assaulting a child of one of the keepers, if that can be so considered; but he has escaped twice, and was caught in an attempt to get through the roof of his cell immediately after his admission.
>
> He has become a powerful and morose young man, determined to escape, or to commit another murder, which he believes would be followed by his execution. He does not hesitate to say that he would prefer being hung to remaining in the asylum without hope of escape.[75]

If the sentiments of Mahso were being accurately reported here then this is another example of a single-minded determination to resist the designs of the British authorities. Escape may have been the preferred option of the inmate but violence is openly considered as a legitimate means of taking on colonial institutionalisation.

Violence as a means of resisting the regimes of the asylums could take many forms. The most direct would be an assault on the superintendent himself, the head of the asylum and the symbol of British authority and control. Dr Crombie at Dacca recounted an episode when 'I was myself the subject of an attack by a lunatic who was sitting quietly weeding in the garden when, without warning, he suddenly sprang to his feet and seized a koodali, and rushed at me with the intention of felling me, but was luckily frustrated.'[76] The resolve to do the British officer damage is also clearly demonstrated in the tenacity of an assault on the superintendent at Patna:

> As I am writing cases, a small, well made man, habitually courteous, and a good weaver, comes up to me, makes an obeisance, says he is quite well and solicits his discharge. Before I can reply, he seizes the pen I have just laid down, that is taken from him, and he makes a dash at my walking stick, and is at once seized by a keeper. That quiet, civil and apparently harmless little man is now a veritable demon; with eyes starting

with rage he tries to seize me, and failing covers me with most violent abuse, and continues to do so as he is being carried off to his cell.[77]

If this account is to be believed then it seems that the Indian inmate is singling out the British medical officer as the target of his anger and abuse even when restrained by the Indian staff.[78] The fact that it is the colonial representative that is made the focus of the patient's outburst of anger makes this a potent demonstration of resistance to colonial authority, especially as the attack is initially directed at the superintendent's pen which was often perceived as a symbol of power.[79]

There are instances where anger and resentment at decisions made by the colonial officers has occasioned violence which was directed at the Indian members of staff as representatives of the colonial order:

> I regret also to record a disastrous out break, attended with loss of life and severe injuries to several of the attendants took place in the Asylum on the 24th of March. An inmate of the Asylum named Keetapai, a non-criminal lunatic who had been under treatment for the past five years ... I had permitted this man to keep a dog; unfortunately a litter of pups were born, and on their growing up they became such a nuisance that I was obliged to order their being disposed of; this was an offence not to be forgiven, And after evidently brooding over it he persuaded a lunatic named Guggur Sing [sic] to join him in attacking the keepers. Keetapai was heard to say 'oh, we are lunatics, we can do what we like and kill them all and nothing will be done to us' ... they simultaneously attacked the warder of the criminal gate, knocked him down and rushed into the garden, attacking every keeper who attempted to oppose them ... the first keeper they met was killed near the entrance of the criminal ward by a fearful blow to the head, they then rushed towards the outer gate when they were met by another burkandaz who they also killed. On hearing the disturbance, Mr Wilson the Deputy Superintendent, who was in his house, rushed into the Asylum to see what was the matter; they met him at the gate and he received some severe blows on the head, but was eventually rescued by the servants and one of the lunatics.[80]

It appears in this example that the decision of the British medical officer resulted in a revenge attack directed not solely at the individual who made the decision but at all of his representatives in the asylum regardless of whether they were Indian or European. The power of the colonial officer to order the lives and the spaces inside the asylum was explicitly contested here by an assault on those who were seen to be obeying his commands and imposing his orders.

Indeed the victim of violent action aimed at resisting the designs

of the asylum regime was not always a representative of that regime. Surgeon-Major Niven at Colaba reported in 1874 that 'one of
the cases, a Parsee, admitted as a private patient under Section VII,
resisted with such determination that when the beef-tea was administered by means of the stomach pump, as soon as the tube
was withdrawn, he ejected the whole contents of the stomach.'[81]
The subject of the violence involved in resisting colonial designs
here was the Indian himself.

Another intriguing example in which it appears that the patient's
own body is a site where the colonial regime was resisted crops up
at the Nagpur asylum in a set of correspondence from 1875. The
matter dealt with was 'the subject of a female lunatic who had
been for several years in the asylum having been delivered of a
child.'[82] That the female portion of the asylum population was routinely segregated from the male in the colonial asylums was
mentioned earlier.[83] This certainly seems to have been the case at
Nagpur where 'the female lunatics are and have been from the first
opening of the asylum lodged, as stated in my report written on
the 19th of June 1868 . . . in a separate building with walled airing
ground distant about 100 yards from the male wards.'[84] Nevertheless the woman had conceived while an inmate of the asylum.
However this came to pass this is certainly an example of someone
at the asylum resisting colonial discipline, as the correct distance
to be preserved by men and women had obviously been ignored.
The '100 yards' was more than a piece of ground; it was a cultural
barrier between the sexes prescribed by colonial power. The child
that was the result of a liaison in the asylum was a physical symbol of resistance to colonial authority as such offspring were
unimaginable in the colonial design for correct relations between
the sexes inside the asylum. Indeed there is the tantalizing suggestion in the evidence that it was the woman herself who had crossed
that '100 yards': 'In the new male ward, in the very furthest room
i.e. furthest from the door, I found a young woman lying on the
ground and two men lying near her. They were the only persons
in this ward at the time.[85]

This statement appears in the report of the Commissioner of Nagpur
who had arrived at the asylum to perform an inspection by chance
in October 1873. It was later confirmed that 'he found a woman
and two men lying asleep in one of the male wards.'[86] It was this
woman who was found to be pregnant the following year in
December. Obviously she did not conceive on this occasion and

the testimony is problematic as it is part of a set of correspondence where officers sought to defend and ruin careers. However
the testimony does not make any suggestion that the woman was
in the male ward because of violence or abduction. This raises the
possibility that her pregnancy was not the result of rape. Indeed, it
could suggest that it was she who had decided to transgress the
boundary prescribed by the British between the females and the
males. Whatever the truth about the child's conception, that conception and that child are vivid demonstrations that even in the
midst of a colonial institution the power of the British to control
and order Indian lives was contested.

Perhaps the most dramatic evidence of resistance strategies involving the body of the individual resisting is in patient suicides.
The summary of one such case reads: 'One lunatic in that asylum
committed suicide by hanging, after having failed in persevering
attempts to starve himself to death.'[87] It transpires in the superintendent's more detailed account that the reason the inmate had
failed to starve himself to death was because 'he had been fed regularly
with the stomach pump.'[88] Again, there are dangers with materials
like this in assuming that the intentions ascribed to Indians were
anything more than the guesses of the authors of the reports. However, if the individual in question had embarked on a period of
self-starvation in order to die and the asylum had responded by
taking control of that individual's body in order to keep him alive,
then the man's decision to take more immediate action to achieve
the state he desired seems to be an instance of self-destruction as
direct resistance to colonial objectives.

Such records of asylum violence though do offer reminders that
not every incident in a colonized country needs contextualizing as
a colonial encounter to explain it. It is perhaps a unique feature of
the asylum records that the medical officer's desire to explain
behavioural patterns in inmates meant that details of their behaviour
before they became the focus of the attention of the colonial authorities are often available. For this reason there is information available
with which it is possible to speculate that incidents, which while
obviously happening in the confines of a colonial institution, do
not necessarily need the colonial context to make them intelligible.
Consider the passage from the Hyderabad superintendent's report:

Restraint has rarely been needed, though we have several very dangerous lunatics in the asylum. One, subject to epileptic fits, murdered a

Bunnia who had insulted him some days previously. For some time the people of the village had dreaded this man, who is very powerful. One day, since he has been in the asylum, he struck down a warder who annoyed him, and unless assistance had been at hand, would have killed him.[89]

The account is obviously difficult to use for reasons associated with doubts about the origins of the various key pieces of information contained within it. However the story still raises the possibility that what appears as an act of resistance to the colonial order, the attack of a patient on a warder, might not have been a clash which needs the colonial relationship in the picture in order to explain it. Of course, in one sense the attack is an act of resistance to the colonial asylum regime, as anything which acted to disrupt or frustrate the aim of the medical officers to have a quiet and orderly institution is necessarily so. But it is not clear that this is an example of a conscious attack on a colonial representative. In other words the bad tempered man is not attacking the warder because the warder is a representative of the colonial order. This could just be an example of a bad tempered man, with a history of reacting violently to abuse, simply doing that, reacting violently to abuse regardless of who or what the abuser could claim to represent.

Consider also the report by Dr Wise of a suicide at Dacca in 1873:

> The death by drowning was a very sad one. Sunia, the wife of one of the keepers, a Hindustani Chetin, was sent to the asylum on the 22nd July with a child five months old, as she had attempted to drown herself in the river. She was dull and melancholic and complained of abdominal pains and giddiness. The expulsion of fourteen lumbrici relieved her of these symptoms. Her affection for her child was most tender. She gradually became more cheerful and of her own accord did a little work. Regret was often expressed that she had tried to commit suicide. On the 18th August, after nursing her child, she went to the well, which is secured with a wooden lid, but in which is an opening 22 inches by 17 through which water is raised. Another lunatic was beside her. Before she could be stopped she had squeezed herself through this opening and before the lid could be removed, she was drowned.[90]

A suicide in a carceral institution is easily construed as an act of resistance as it represents the ultimate form of escape when other means of liberation are denied. However the history included in this case suggests that simply because a decision is made in the colonial context it is not to be assumed that that context provides all the information with which to understand that decision. The woman's decision to kill herself might be seen in hindsight as an act of resistance to the colonial regime as any act which denies that regime the power to decide an individual's fate is contesting the rights claimed by that regime. Yet a reading sympathetic to the woman in the superintendent's account would have it that it was the personal pain that haunted her long before she was incarcerated in the asylum which drove her to repeatedly attempt self-destruction. It just so happened that she was a colonial inmate at the time she finally succeeded in taking her own life.

While all those Indians in the asylum were subjects of colonial power, most had ended up there as a result of the operations of the colonial state and were fed, cleaned, and treated according to colonial instructions, it must not be assumed that all of their decisions can be related back to that position of subjection. Some allowance should be made for the fact that in many instances even those Indians confined in that most colonial of contexts, the carceral institution, could make decisions about their own interaction with the world without regard for their position as subjects of colonial power.

It must not be assumed however that resistance was typical of the patients inside the asylums. In certain cases it appears that the asylum environment may have offered a protected space where there was scope for finding new roles and building new relationships. The following account comes from the case note of Neroo:

> This boy is a speechless, slavering idiot. Can scarcely give intimation to be led away to answer the calls of nature. Makes a kind of whining noise when angry. Suffered once from fever and dysentery. General health now fairly good, altho' limbs are weak. He has a frequent rocking motion but pays no attention to what passes around him. He was brought from the Almshouse. No history or trace of parents or relations.
>
> There is no change whatever in this boy except that he has attached himself to one of the lunatic inmates who has taught him to feed himself. General health good.[91]

It would seem that quite independent of the asylum regime and the staff of the institution the boy's levels of interaction with the world had increased and he had developed skills which he had given little evidence of ever having possessed before. This was due to a friendship that had developed between inmates in this colonial space apparently without the intervention or encouragement of anyone but the individuals involved. Of interest for similar reasons is the case of Phoola who 'took a great fancy to a newly born infant whose mother a lunatic, would not look at it. Kept it continually on her knee + finally put it to her own breast, whence in three or four days milk actually flowed.'[92] As was discussed earlier the reasons for this information being included on a case note are tied up in the power relations of the medical and colonial gaze. However, if the fact that a woman has decided to nurture an unwanted child is believed then this could be an interesting instance of an Indian setting out to satisfy her own desires and act according to her perceptions and agendas regardless of the colonial setting of the asylum and its regimen.

While these people were building new relationships others found themselves new roles in life within the asylum which gave them some satisfaction. Of one inmate it was said, 'he may be said to have a kind disposition, as evinced in his attention to the sick – and his great boast was that he had cured some of the patients after they had been given up by the Native Doctor and myself.'[93] Curiously the superintendent makes no attempt to rebut the boast so there remains the image of a patient carving out a function for himself in the asylum as a carer for the weak and the ill given up as a lost cause by the institution.

Indeed it should be pointed out that some inmates may even have actively endorsed the regime of the colonial institution. 'There are several who would not leave the Asylum even if permitted to do so and during the past year three of the discharged insanes have come back begging to be re-admitted. One of the three walked forty miles from the Civil Station of Barh. As might be expected, such men are somewhat silly, and they miss the kind care and attention to their wants when they go to their houses',[94] noted the superintendent at Dullunda. In a similar vein the medical officer at Poona related the fact that in 1876

> the re-admission was a native of Hindustan upwards of a thousand miles from the asylum. He had been discharged in the early part of the year, his brother having come to take him home; he had money of his own. After some months not being happy he left without telling any of his friends, with only a few rupees in his pockets and came back to the asylum, asking to be re-admitted.[95]

It would seem that as part of their personal survival strategies these patients were opting for the asylum regime over a struggle with life in the environment outside of the carceral walls.

Perhaps most important of all it must be remembered that the majority of those admitted to the colonial asylum did not get pregnant, did not murder or attack anyone and did not even bother to hurl a word or two of abuse. More typical than the patients who acted in such ways, or indeed than those who actively sought to carve out roles or relationships in the asylum or to secure a permanent berth there were those whose case notes read like that of Sunkura:

> Sunkura alias Hungra. M. Dementia. Mussul. beggar. 25. 21 Novr.1861. Admitted from the Lucknow Havalabee. He was obstreperous + very incoherent in his speech on admission. For several months little improvement has appeared, but for the last 2 months he has been quiet + well conducted and has worked steadily in the garden. He is now sufficiently well to be discharged.[96]

Far from resisting the asylum regime Sunkura calms down after a period of upset or anger and sets about doing what is expected of him as a patient in a mental institution. He gives noone any trouble, does his work and secures his release.

Conclusion

The asylum was an alien place in Indian society and was in every way implicated in the power relations of colonialism. The people who found themselves inmates of the institution were, with the exceptions mentioned in Chapter 5, incarcerated because the colonial authorities viewed them as potential sources of disruption. The regime designed for them once incarcerated envisioned treating their bodies and their minds so that they would become models of utility for the colonial design, as ordered, self-regulating and productive individuals. Colonial power put them in the asylum and would transform them.

Their responses to being placed in this most colonial of milieus are extremely important then as 'resistance even at its most ambiguous . . . highlights the presence and play of power in most forms of relationship and activity.'[97] Indeed, the responses of individuals isolated in these institutions seems to be just the place to examine the actions and reactions of colonial subjects as these are just the sort of place to which the contemporary historian is being directed in search of resistances, Rosalind O'Hanlon for one urging that 'we should look for resistances of a different kind: dispersed in fields we do not conventionally associate with the political.'[98]

What is apparent then is that in the asylum there were many

acts of resistance but acts of the kind that James Scott has described as, 'individual and often anonymous.'[99] In one sense many of the acts described have been acts of resistance to the colonial order of the asylum be they intended as such or not. The decision to attack the European superintendent of the asylum may be seen as a moment when colonial authority was overtly contested as might the decision to refuse to do more than the bare minimum at work or to carry out the full range of duties expected by the colonial authority. Yet the decision to have sexual intercourse in the ward of the opposite sex, or the urge to commit suicide while an inmate, may also be seen as acts of resistance to colonial power simply because they acted to upset specifically designed colonial orders.

It is just as important to remember that not all responses to colonial power can be characterized as resistance. Often Indians worked hard to make the regimes of colonialism work although here it must be remembered that they did so not because they were subjected by colonial power but because they had their own agendas to pursue in which the opportunities presented by colonialism were welcomed as the means to an end.

Perhaps most significant of all though is the fact that it appears that not all actions in the colonial context, even one as overtly disciplinary as a carceral institution, can be related to that context. What drove many of the people described in this chapter appear to have been demons and desires, pain or pressures which were powerful but the origins of which predated entry into the asylum. As such the colonial medical context does not provide all of the explanations for many of the acts, even if those acts may be retrospectively read as resistance simply because they frustrated the designs of the asylums. Indeed, it may well be that in explaining the suicidal mother, or the ongoing violence of the angry man the colonial medical context provides no information about why these people were acting in such ways. To satisfactorily understand what drove them to behave in such ways it might be the case that the colonial medical context is utterly irrelevant as these people would have behaved in the same way no matter what the context such was the power of their pain. This reminds the historian not to shade colonial power into accounts of Indian actions in the nineteenth century on the assumption that it was significant rather than on the evidence that it was so. This will be more fully discussed in the conclusion.

Conclusion: Knowledge, Power and Agency

All these folk are saying, 'It was plague. We've had the plague here'.
You'd almost think they expected to be given medals for it. But what
does that mean – 'plague'? Just life, no more than that.[1]

The period 1857 to 1880 began with considerable ambitions for
those that the British considered to be lunatic in British India and
ended in asylum closures and special investigations into the expense of providing such institutions. For example, in 1862 there
was an exchange of correspondence between the North-Western
Provinces and the Government of India about a survey that the
Inspector-General of Prisons had organized. After canvassing the
District Officers of the area he estimated the total number of lunatics in the NWP:

> Dr Clark's own conviction resulting from his own investigation is that
> there are 1250 cases to be provided for. Of this 328 can be sent to
> Bareilly and 328 to Benares so that there are still 600 candidates for
> admission to the proposed asylum.[2]

His plan was to house *all* those considered 'lunatic' in institutions
to be provided for the purpose, even the '957 . . . said to be taken
care of by their friends, a circumstance which I think very doubtful at least, the amount of care bestowed upon them must, I fear,
be very small indeed.'[3]

By the end of the 1870s such ambitions would have been un-
thinkable. Typical of the period was the Bengal Medical Expenditure
(O'Kinealy) Committee of 1878/9[4] which devoted a separate section of its report to the lunatic asylums of the area. The differing
costs of the patients in each asylum, the diverse dieting arrangements

and associated expenditure and the varying commitment of each superintendent to profitable manufacturing were all investigated as the cost of providing such facilities began to be felt as a burden. With the closure of the Moydapore asylum in 1877 and the Hazaribagh asylum in 1879 the last years of the 1870s signalled an end to the burst of energy which had more than doubled in two decades the number of asylums that the British had managed to get up and running by 1858.

An investigation of this burst of energy has implications for a number of current debates within the history of medicine and also within the controversies about the nature of colonial encounters and colonial experiences. Many historians of colonial contexts share with historians of medicine a concern about the nature of the knowledge generated within the systems that they investigate. It is worth emphasizing then that this study concurs with the conclusion that, 'patient records are surviving artefacts of the interaction between physicians and their patients in which individual personality, cultural assumptions, social status, bureaucratic expediency, and the reality of power relationships are expressed.'[5] Documents such as the case notes at the Lucknow asylum are sites where ideas and identities were constructed, ideas and identities produced from within a range of discourses such as colonial difference, medical professionalism, modern masculinity and so on. Examining these sources reveals much about the way in which those writing the documents thought about themselves, about their work in India and about the Indians that they were dealing with. They reveal little however of the minds of which they claimed to be a record, in other words these psychiatric records can tell the historian nothing reliable about the mentalities of the patients who it was claimed were the subjects of the case notes.

These medical documents then were works of the imagination, of the imaginations of British male medical officers who worked in India in the high colonial period. That these imaginations survive in documentary form is a reflection of the power relations of the period, as the British had the power to watch and to write about the Indians admitted to the colonial institutions. But the study of the development within the Government of India of a concern about cannabis use among the Indian population demonstrates how the generation of knowledge within the government of the colonizers was more than simply an exercise in whimsy. The ideas and identities constructed in the asylum records did not remain isolated in the archives of the institutions where they were set down on paper. The asylum, like the prison and the army barrack,[6] was one of the few points where the British administration came into regular and controlled close contact with samples of the Indian population. British administrators fretted about their lack of knowledge of Indian societies and communities: 'Until some . . . network of enquiry is skilfully spread abroad the country we shall never be in a position to judge what is naturally going on in the inner life and domestic concerns of the teeming population of India.'[7]

As such, the information that was available to them became all the more important and the asylum records were seized upon by civil administrators and government officials as rare glimpses of an otherwise inscrutable population which nevertheless it was their task to reorder and govern. In this way the knowledge generated at the asylum, that product of the imaginings of the medical officers at the asylums and the expedients of Indian officials assumed wider significance. The meta-language of statistics and the information gathering systems of colonialism meant that the way the asylum superintendent saw his patients quickly became a way that colonial government in general saw the Indian population as a whole.

Indeed, investigating imagined human types like the 'ganja-smoker' and the formulation of social problems like 'cannabis use' acts as a reminder that exposing 'produced' knowledge is not just an arid exercise in tracing the archaeology of governmental categories or the information network of a modern regime. Such an investigation leads directly to lived experience as power was exercised on the basis of the knowledge produced at the asylum. Men were incarcerated and customs or habits demonized and criminalized by the regime in India because of the way the superintendent saw his patients and the way the colonial system was geared to collate and disseminate his observations.

The asylum was of course fully implicated in the power relations of colonial India as it was placed in tandem with larger British projects to drill or discipline the Indian population by removing the troublesome and the unproductive. The asylum was also designed to function on the micro-level as the internal regime at the asylums was to discipline those individuals removed from Indian society. This regime was intended to act upon the bodies and minds of those incarcerated so that ordered and productive individuals would be created from what the British perceived as the jumbled and chaotic Indian. In the asylums of British India then it is possible to see where medical techniques and technologies came to serve the interests of colonial administrators and of colonial projects, just as medical power has been accused of serving the ambitions of modern government in Europe. But it is important to note that this convergence of the medical and the colonial was not axiomatic, and that there are examples from cases involving lunatics in which medical power and the objectives of colonial government in India operated in conflict. The following is an account of the case of Abdulla, a convict at Port Blair:

> After his arrival he refused altogether to work and he was impertinent and excited when spoken to. I therefore sent him before the 3rd medical officer for examination and opinion as to mental condition. That officer replied that in his opinion the man was suffering from mental aberration. I then wrote to the officer in charge Northern District recommending the man for transfer to the Haddo Lunatic Asylum and pointing out that the Jail was not a proper place for a man in his condition.
>
> Before submission of the recommendation to the Chief Commissioner the matter was referred to the senior medical officer who examined the man and stated that in his opinion the convict was only feigning madness.
>
> A copy of his memo being sent to me, I then sentenced the man to six stripes with a rattan. The 3rd medical officer, however, being of opinion that he is insane declines to pass him for that punishment.[8]

The colonial officer was eager to exercise disciplinary power in this example and he intended to punish the man's body in order to manage his behaviour. However the power of the medical judgement as an estimation of human competence acted to frustrate those disciplinary designs. The senior medical officer eventually concurred with the opinion of his junior colleague and the convict was sent to the asylum untouched by the colonial rattan.

If this example can be used to demonstrate that medical power did not always serve the purposes of colonial government it also stands as a reminder about the importance of the local, contingent nature of decision making in British India. The case is an example where there was no clear and well-defined procedure and the deliberation of a wavering senior medical officer caught between two opposing decisions determined the outcome. The importance of the local and contingent is a theme which has developed throughout this book. It is all very well to trace in the documents the ideas, intentions and objectives of colonial officials and the elaborate schemes that they concocted for managing India. But it must be remembered when reading these that these are all schemes on paper and that there is no guarantee that the objectives or systems were ever realized. When considering admissions for example it was shown that those who were incarcerated in the asylums fell into broad categories but that not all of those who fell into those broad categories were incarcerated in the asylums. Localized and contingent factors, like the presence of witnesses or the agendas of local officials, were what acted to single out those who were to become asylum inmates.

Similarly, both chapters in which the responses of Indians around and inside the asylum were considered showed that Indians had a range of objectives and agendas in interacting with the asylums. These were often highly individualized interactions which again emphasize the essentially local and specific nature of encounters between the British and Indians. The objectives and interactions of Indians in these encounters often decided the outcome of these encounters, in other words it was Indians resisting or Indians facilitating colonial designs which could determine whether British systems worked or whether British objectives were met.

Such observations are important as rejoinders to those who still have a somewhat Fanonian vision of the colonial encounter where, 'this encounter was framed by and riddled in the fundamental fact about both colonialism and Orientalism: domination.'[9] The colonizers did not dominate but desired to dominate and the instances where their projects were disrupted and contested emphasize that their domination remained fantasy rather than 'fact' and remained well short of 'hegemonic.'

They are also important as rejoinders to those who have rather Foucauldian visions of asylums and other medical institutions. Michel Foucault's vision of such institutions and their regimes tended to be expressed in very absolute terms. As has already been stated, for Foucault the asylum was 'A religious domain without religion, a domain of pure morality, of ethical uniformity... an instrument of moral uniformity and of social denunciation.'[10] The frustration of the asylum regime by the Indian staff and the resistance offered by the patients shows that while the asylum may have been established and intended as an instrument of 'moral uniformity', in reality it rarely functioned as such. The patients who seem to be acting without regard to their environment are perhaps the most interesting here. Those who sneaked off for sex or who formed friendships with other patients show that within the asylum there was in practice considerable space for pursuing agendas arrived at independently of the designs of the asylum. In short, in the colonial medical institution, neither colonial power or medical power was absolute or dominant.

It is important to remember however that in key respects many such moments of resistance to colonial and institutional power were no such thing. The decision to assault, have sex or self-immolate was often taken without regard to the colonial or institutional context despite the setting being the colonial institution. Such decisions may well have resulted in the frustration of colonial and medical designs but they were never intended to have such an impact. Indeed, they may well have been intended as acts of resistance, but not resistance to colonial or medical power. The woman's suicide after the birth of her child could be placed in the context of contesting patriarchal culture, while the man's violent reactions to insult might just as easily be placed in the context of local standards of status and honour. Whatever is correct, the evidence certainly suggests that these individuals were often pursuing agendas which were arrived at before they became inmates of the asylum and subjects of colonial and medical power.

Similarly it is rather one dimensional to see those Indians in the asylum who were cooperating with the colonial order, the attendants who made the asylum tick or the patients who carved out roles in the institution which guaranteed its smooth running as collaborators oppressed by colonial power or taken in by its hegemonic power. It seems more likely in this study that they were not doing the bidding of the colonizer because they were purely subjects of colonial power. Rather, the opportunity presented by the colonial system for employment, security, enrichment and so on provided a way for them to pursue or realize their own agendas which had been arrived at largely without reference to colonial designs. These agendas would have included personal comfort or advancement, family income and security and so on. In other words these would have been agendas which may have been determined, and were no doubt in the process of being transformed and determined at the moment of decision, by reference to a range of cultural systems, which may sometimes indeed have included the colonial but which may also have included the familial, the patriarchal, the communal and so on. In this sense then Nicholas Thomas is correct to point out that the habitual relating of the actions of indigenous peoples to the colonial context just because they occur in that context 'excludes the possibility that "natives" often had relatively autonomous representations and agendas that might have been deaf to the enunciations of colonialism.'[11]

Indeed, even those examples given in previous chapters where the action of an individual seems directly linked to the colonial presence, and that colonial presence seems to be the essential factor in the decision to act in that way, cannot be assumed to be as they appear. Although much of the work in this project has sought to deconstruct the 'lunatic' status of those deemed so by the British, the possibility that some of those so called did experience mental states which would be popularly called 'madness' raises intriguing possibilities. The fact that certain individuals imagined themselves kings, princes or even deities when they appear not to have been makes their agendas an extremely difficult subject upon which to speculate. It is true that these people would have had agendas, but not ones which were related to anything that a good social scientist would be able to discover such as gender, social status, position in the colonial hierarchy and so on. In other words these people remind us that there is the possibility of highly individualized decision making which may have very little to do with those aspects of the universe that a historian or sociologist would be able to pick out of a historical document.

This issue of highly individualized decision making raises the debates about individual agency in society, debates recently described as 'central to much recent work in both anthropology and history.'[12] As Dirks, Eley and Ortner described in Chapter 6, the search has been on for 'a subject who is at once culturally and historically constructed, yet from a political perspective, we would wish this subject to be capable of acting in some sense "autonomously", not simply in conformity to dominant cultural norms and rules.'[13] It has been demonstrated in many of the examples included in this study that individuals can be capable of novel and creative actions which serve to disrupt and frustrate the systems that seek to subject them. In other words the 'lunatic' actions of certain individuals simply serve to demonstrate *in extremis* the power of the individual to act without regard to the social and cultural context in which they are found. Here are examples of 'the autonomous actor', capable of acting without conformity to dominant cultural norms and rules.

This is not to resurrect the figure of Western humanism which Rosalind O'Hanlon has called, 'the self-originating, self-determining individual, who is at once a subject in his possession of a sovereign consciousness whose defining quality is reason and an agent in his power of freedom.'[14] Rather it is to emphasize a point that she makes elsewhere that, 'power takes effect: as a play of forces which continually moves across and bursts through our efforts to establish coherent fields of activity.'[15]

If she had said 'power(s)' she would have been more accurate. The only factor mentioned in Chapter 6 when trying to explain these highly individualized actions was physiological illness, which acts to alter brain structures and therefore to alter brain functioning. Alongside this might be added genetic dispositions and the functioning of body chemistry. Such factors, invisible to the historian or anthropologist, begin to explain how individuals can be seen to be acting without regard to cultural rules or norms in certain circumstances but without having to assign to individuals the 'sovereign will' of the humanist project. The complex interplay of genetics, physiological chemistry and disease within each body serves to create individuals in the most literal sense of the word, unique units with distinct sets of characteristics. The 'lunatic' actions of some of the cases are better described as instances where the uniqueness of the individual is demonstrated and where it was experienced as unpredictability or non-conformity by systems of government which acted to discredit and punish that uniqueness.

On this interpretation then the individual can be an agent in society and history and can act in unique and creative ways outside of the dictates of systems of cultural, social and political power. The individual is not doing so as he/she is the possessor of an innate and mysterious will, rather because he/she is the subject of powers which are invisible to the social scientist, the powers of genetics, body chemistry, disease and so on. Here then is the individual who acts autonomously of social and cultural rules and norms. However this is not an individual who is truly independent of all 'power', as those moments when he/she is disrupting the power of social rules and norms are moments when he/she is governed by the power of his/her individual genes, hormones, illnesses and so on.

This of course is overstating the case as no example will ever be that clear cut as a range of impulses and pressures will lay behind any one action. The point of the overstatement is to make clear that many of these impulses and pressures come from a source outside of that of the structures of social and cultural power. Many of these impulses and pressures come from within the individual and as such the individual can properly be seen as an agent in society and history.

The implications of this for the broader themes of this study is that in asylums individuals can be spotted displaying an utter disregard for the power of colonial government and of Western medicine despite the fact that they are in the midst of an institution designed to be 'total.' On this account it might be said that colonial power, medical power or indeed, the power of any other social and cultural systems, of patriarchy, religion, of class, caste and so on is never absolute, as indeed the power of genes, hormones or diseases and so on is never absolute.

Power is everywhere and behind every action and sometimes the historian or the social scientist attempts to name it, as colonial power or patriarchal power or medical power or the power of hormones, or genetics and so on. Yet it is just power, and attaching too much significance to naming it at any one moment obscures this fact. Colonial power is not really colonial power, medical power is not really medical power and so on. Like the plague in the Camus novel they are just power. And that is, after all, 'just life, no more than that.'

Appendix: Asylums Operating in the Period 1857–1880

These institutions are arranged by administration and by alphabetical order. The date in the bracket is included if the asylum has been positively identified as founded in this period.

ASSAM	Tezpore (1876)
	Berhampore (1874)
	Cuttack (1864)
	Dullunda
BENGAL	Dacca
	Hazaribagh (1876)
	Moydapore
	Patna
	Ahmedabad (1862)
	Colaba
BOMBAY	Dharwar
	Hyderabad (c.1871)
	Poona (1867)
BURMA	Rangoon (1870)
CENTRAL PROVINCES	Jubbulpore (c.1867)
	Nagpur (1864)*
HYDERABAD ASSIGNED DISTRICTS	Amraoti (1877)
	Calicut
MADRAS	Madras
	Vizagapatam (1863)*
	Agra (1869)
NORTH-WESTERN PROVINCES	Bareilly (1862)*
	Benares
OUDH	Lucknow (1859)

PUNJAB   Delhi (1867)
                                         Lahore

Unless otherwise stated the date for the opening of the asylum was found
in the records of the period.

* Date available in S. Sharma, *Mental Hospitals in India* (Directorate General
of Health Services, New Delhi, 1990).

Notes

Introduction

1 Civ.Surg.Rangoon to IMDBurma 15 January 1877, GOI (Medical) Procs October 1877, 18–20B.
2 J. Scott, *Weapons of the Weak: everyday forms of peasant resistance* (Yale University Press New Haven 1985).
3 M. Foucault, *The Birth of the Clinic: an archaeology of medical perception* (Tavistock London 1973), p. 196.
4 N. Fairclough, *Critical Discourse Analysis: the critical study of language* (Longman London 1995), p. 6.
5 R. Guha, 'The Prose of Counter-Insurgency', in R. Guha, *Subaltern Studies II* (Oxford University Press New Delhi 1983), p. 4.
6 Ibid., p. 15.
7 S. Amin, 'Approver's Testimony, Judicial Discourse: the case of Chauri Chaura', in R. Guha, *Subaltern Studies V* (Oxford University Press New Delhi 1987), p. 167.
8 Ibid., p. 198.
9 R. MacLeod and M. Lewis (eds), 'Introduction', in *Disease, Medicine and Empire: perspectives on western medicine and the experience of European expansion* (Routledge London 1988), p. 1.
10 J. Matthews, *Good and Mad Women: the historical construction of femininity in twentieth-century Australia* (Allen and Unwin St. Leonards 1984), pp. 25–8.
11 C. Coleborne, 'Gender and the patient case-book in the lunatic asylum in colonial Victoria (Australia)', presented to the Society for the Social History of Medicine *Medicine and the Colonies Conference* (Oxford 1996), p. 2.
12 M. Foucault (translated by R. Howard), *Madness and Civilization: a history of insanity in the Age of Reason* (Routledge London 1989).
13 'This strange republic of the good which is imposed by force on all those suspected of belonging to evil', in ibid., p. 61.
14 Ibid., p. 62.
15 Ibid., p. 276.
16 Ibid., p. 259.

17 A. Scull, 'Humanitarianism or Control? Some observations on the historiography of Anglo-American psychiatry', in S. Cohen and A. Scull (eds), *Social Control and the State* (Basil Blackwell Oxford 1985), p. 134.

18 E. Showalter, *The Female Malady: women, madness and English culture 1830–1980* (Virago London 1987), p. 18.

19 Y. Ripa, *Women and Madness: the incarceration of women in nineteenth-century France* (Polity Press Cambridge 1990), p. 3.

20 Ibid., pp. 160–1.

21 N. Rose, *The Psychological Complex: psychology, politics and society in England 1869–1939* (Routledge London 1985), p. 227.

22 F. Fanon, 'Medicine and Colonialism', in J. Ehrenreich (ed.), *The Cultural Crisis of Modern Medicine* (Monthly Review Press New York 1978), p. 229.

23 R. MacLeod, 'Introduction', p. 2; see also D. Arnold, 'Introduction', in D. Arnold (ed.), *Imperial Medicine and Indigenous Societies* (Oxford University Press New Delhi 1988), p. 18.

24 M. Harrison, *Public Health in British India: Anglo-Indian preventive medicine 1859–1914* (Cambridge University Press Cambridge 1994), pp. 117–38; M. Lyons, *The Colonial Disease: a social history of sleeping sickness in northern Zaire 1900–1940* (Cambridge University Press Cambridge 1992).

25 R. Ileto, 'Cholera and the origins of the American sanitary order in the Philippines', in D. Arnold (ed.), *Imperial Medicine*; D. Arnold, *Colonizing the Body: state medicine and epidemic disease in nineteenth-century India* (Oxford University Press New Delhi 1993), pp. 200–39.

26 V. Oldenburg, *The Making of Colonial Lucknow 1856–1877* (Princeton University Press Princeton 1984), pp. 96–144.

27 C. Coleborne, 'Legislating lunacy and the body of the female lunatic', in D. Kirkby (ed.), *Sex, Power and Justice: historical perspectives on law in Australia* (Oxford University Press Melbourne 1995), p. 95.

28 S. Swartz, 'The Black Insane in the Cape 1891–1920', in *Journal of Southern African Studies* 21, 1995.

29 Y. Lee, 'Lunatics and Lunatic Asylums in early Singapore 1819–1869', in *Medical History* 19, 1973, p. 34.

30 W. Ernst, *Mad Tales from the Raj: the European insane in British India 1800–1858* (Routledge London 1991), pp. 164–73.

31. A. Yang, *Crime and Criminality in British India* (University of Arizona Press Tucson 1985); D. Arnold, *Police Power and Colonial Rule: Madras 1859–1947* (Oxford University Press New Delhi 1986); D. Arnold, 'The Colonial Prison: power, knowledge and penology in nineteenth-century India', in D. Arnold and D. Hardiman (eds), *Subaltern Studies VIII* (Oxford University Press New Delhi 1994).

32 R. Porter, *A Social History of Madness: stories of the insane* (Weidenfeld and Nicolson London 1987), p. 231.

33 J. Mattlock, *Scenes of Seduction: prostitution, hysteria and reading difference in nineteenth-century France* (Columbia University Press New York 1994), p. 185.

34 Y. Ripa, *Women and Madness*, p. 138.

35 C. Warsh, 'Moments of Unreason: the practice of Canadian psychiatry and the Homewood retreat 1883–1923', quoted in C. Coleborne, *Resistances*

and the negotiation of 'mad' identities (unpublished paper), p. 5.

36 P. Chesler, *Women and Madness* (Allen Lane London 1984), p. 16.
37 R. Guha, 'On Some Aspects of the Historiography of Colonial India', in R. Guha (ed.), *Subaltern Studies I* (Oxford University Press New Delhi 1982), p. 4.
38 N. Thomas, *Colonialism's Culture: anthropology, travel and government* (Polity Press Oxford 1994), p. 57.
39 *Report on the Asylums, Vaccination and Dispensaries in Bengal, 1868–1873*, p. 13.
40 Case Book IA, patient no. 163, admitted 3 April 1865: 'chumar' means leatherworker.
41 Case Book IA, patient no. 158, admitted 28 February 1865: 'ahir' means herdsman.
42 Chief Commissioner to Gvt.Bengal in Bengal (Military) 3 April 1795.
43 Letters received from Bengal 14 May 1795, paragraph 27.
44 *Annual Report on the Insane Asylums in Bengal for the Year 1879*, p. 1.
45 *Asylums in Bengal for the Year 1877*, p. 29.
46 See Appendix.
47 *Asylums in Bengal for the Year 1875*, p. 17.
48 *Annual Administration and Progress Report on the Insane Asylums in the Bombay Presidency for the Year 1874–5*, pp. 30–3.
49 Ibid.
50 *Asylums in the Bombay Presidency for the Year 1880* p. 8.
51 *Asylums in the Bombay Presidency for the Year 1900*, p. 8.
52 *Annual Report of the Three Lunatic Asylums in the Madras Presidency during the Year 1877–8*, p. 33.
53 *Asylums in the Madras Presidency during the Year 1879–80*, p. 29.
54 *Asylums in the Madras Presidency during the Year 1890*, p. 10.
55 *Asylums in the Madras Presidency during the Year 1900*, p. 20.
56 Ibid.
57 *Annual Report of the Insane Asylums in Bengal for the Year 1875*, p. 28.
58 *Asylums in Bengal for the Year 1890*, p. 2.
59 *Asylums in Bengal for the Year 1900*, p. 2.
60 This does not include the Lucknow Asylum and the three Asylums in the North-Western Provinces, for which figures are not available.

1 The Asylum Archive: the Production of Knowledge at the Colonial Asylum

1 *Annual Report on the Insane Asylums in Bengal for the Year 1871*, p. 83.
2 IGH.IMD to GOI 6 January 1873, GOI (Public) Procs January 1873, 529A.
3 See GOI (Medical) Procs September 1874, 60–3A.
4 For example see the *Report on the Lunatic Asylums in the Central Provinces for the Year 1874* (that was prepared and submitted in 1875). This was the year that the Resolution was passed, but the summary for Nagpur includes ten tables, Jubbulpore eleven.
5 For studies of national asylum histories see for example, D. Rothman,

The Discovery of the Asylum: social order and disorder in the New Republic (Little Brown Boston 1971); G. Grob, *Mental Institutions in America: social policy to 1875* (NY Free Press New York 1973); A. Scull, *The Most Solitary of Afflictions: madness and society in Britain, 1700–1900* (Yale University Press London 1993); M. Finnane, *Insanity and the Insane in post-Famine Ireland* (Croom Helm London 1981); S. Garton, *Medicine and Madness: a social history of insanity in New South Wales, 1880–1940* (New South Wales University Press Kensington NSW 1988); R. Castel, *The Regulation of Madness: the origins of incarceration in France* (Polity Press Oxford 1988). Case studies of individual institutions include, R. Hunter and I. MacAlpine, *Psychiatry for the Poor. 1851 Colney Hatch Asylum-Friern Hospital 1973: a medical and social history* (Dawsons Folkestone 1974); N. Tomes, *A Generous Confidence: Thomas Story Kirkbride and the Art of Asylum Keeping, 1840–1883* (Cambridge University Press Cambridge 1985); A. Digby, *Madness, Morality and Medicine: a study of the York Retreat, 1796–1914* (Cambridge University Press Cambridge 1985; E. Dwyer, *Homes for the Mad: life inside two nineteenth century asylums* (Rutgers University Press New Brunswick 1987); E. Malcolm, *Swift's Hospital: a story of St. Patrick's Hospital, Dublin 1746–1989* (Gill and Macmillan Dublin 1989); C. MacKenzie, *Psychiatry for the Rich: a history of the Private Ticehurst Asylum, 1792–1917* (Routledge London 1992).

6 See A. Digby, *Madness, Morality and Medicine*; R. Hunter and I. MacAlpine, *Psychiatry for the Poor*; N. Tomes, *A Generous Confidence*; S. Short, *Victorian Lunacy: Richard M. Bucke and the Practice of late Nineteenth-century Psychiatry* (Cambridge University Press Cambridge 1986).

7 See T. Turner, 'Schizophrenia as a Permanent Problem', *History of Psychiatry*, 3, 1992; E. Renvoize and A. Beveridge, 'Mental Illness and the late Victorians: a study of patients admitted to three asylums in York 1880–1884', in *Psychological Medicine*, 19, 1989; R. Persaud, 'A comparison of symptoms recorded from the same patients by an asylum doctor and a "Constant Observer" in 1823: the implications for theories about psychological illness in history', in *History of Psychiatry*, 3, 1992.

8 It has been argued that statistics are a productive medium which does no more than create new identities rather than transparently relate existing ones. As such it is not at all clear that an exercise in statistical compilation is desirable if the objective is to get an accurate picture of a group or population. See for example, I. Hacking, 'Making Up People', in T. Heller, M. Sosna and D. Wellerby (eds), *Reconstructing Individualism: autonomy, individuality and the self in Western thought* (Stanford University Press Stanford 1986); B. Cohn, 'The Census, Social Structure and Objectification in South India', in B.Cohn (ed.), *An Anthropologist among the Historians and Other Essays* (Oxford University Press 1987).

9 *Annual Report on the Lunatic Asylums in the Madras Presidency during the Year 1877–78*, p. 5.

10 Case Book IA, patient no. 110, admitted 30 May 1861.

11 Case Book IV, patient no. 54, admitted 31 August 1868.

12 Case Book II, patient no. 106, admitted 10 June 1864.

13 *Annual Administration and Progress Report on the Insane Asylums in the Bombay Presidency for the Year 1873–4*, p. 6.

14 Robertson Milne-Collection LHB7/58/2 (20).

15 For another consideration of the difficulties experienced by the British in recording the age of Indians see T. Albarn, 'Age and Empire in the Indian Census, 1871–1931', in *Journal of Interdisciplinary History*, xxx, 1999.

16 J. Wise, 'General Paralysis of the Insane', in *Indian Medical Gazette*, iv, 1869.

17 Asylums in Bengal for the Year 1867, p. 60.

18 A. Beveridge, 'Madness in Victorian Edinburgh: a study of patients admitted to the Royal Edinburgh Asylum under Thomas Clouston 1873–1908, Part II', in *History of Psychiatry*, 6, 1995, p. 134.

19 Ibid., p. 135.

20 Ibid.

21 A. Digby, *Madness, Morality and Medicine*, p. 136.

22 *Asylums in Bengal for the Year 1885*, p. 3.

23 *Asylums in Bengal for the Year 1867*, p. 42: The five headings referred to here are moral insanity, monomania, mania (acute and chronic) and amentia.

24 *Asylums in the Central Provinces for the Year 1878*, p. 2.

25 R. Persaud, 'The Reporting of Psychiatric Symptoms in History: the memorandum book of Samuel Coates 1785–1925', in *History of Psychiatry*, 4, 1993, p. 510.

26 T. Turner, 'Schizophrenia as a Permanent Problem', p. 427

27 R. Parker, A. Dutta, R. Barnes and T. Fleet, 'County of Lancaster Asylum, Rainhill: 100 years ago and now', in *History of Psychiatry*, 4, 1993, p. 100.

28 A. Beveridge, 'Madness in Victorian Edinburgh, Part II', p. 143.

29 R. Persaud, 'A comparison of symptoms', p. 93.

30 T. Turner, 'Schizophrenia as a Permanent Problem', p. 428.

31 R. Parker *et al.*, 'County of Lancaster Asylum, Rainhill', p. 105.

32 H. White, *Tropics of Discourse: essays in cultural criticism* (Johns Hopkins University Press Baltimore 1978), p. 232.

33 N. Fairclough, *Critical Discourse Analysis: the critical study of language* (Longman London 1995), p. 6.

34 See for example G. Risse and J. Warner, 'Reconstructing Clinical Activities: patient records and medical history', in *Social History of Medicine*, 5, 1992; P. Wright and A. Treacher (eds), *The Problem of Medical Knowledge: examining the social construction of medicine* (Edinburgh University Press Edinburgh 1982).

35 L. Jordanova, 'The Social Construction of Medical Knowledge', in *Social History of Medicine*, 8, 1995, p. 362.

36 J. Matthews, *Good and Mad Women: the historical construction of femininity in twentieth century Australia* (Allen and Unwin St. Leonards 1984), p. 28.

37 C. Coleborne, '"She does her hair up fantastically": the production of femininity in patient case books of the lunatic asylum in 1860s Victoria', in J. Long (ed.), *Forging Identities: bodies, gender and feminist history*

(University of Western Australia Press Nedlands 1997), p. 48.

38   R. Guha, 'The Prose of Counter-Insurgency', in R. Guha, *Subaltern Studies II* (Oxford University Press New Delhi 1983), p. 15.

39   S. Swartz, 'Changing Diagnoses in Valkenberg Asylum, Cape Colony 1891–1920', in *History of Psychiatry*, 6, 1995.

40   J. Andrews, 'Case Notes, Case Histories, and the Patient's Experience of Insanity at Gartnavel Royal Asylum, Glasgow, in the Nineteenth Century', in *Social History of Medicine*, 11, 1998, p. 266.

41   Case Book IA, patient no. 194, admitted 13 May 1862.

42   Case Book IA, patient no. 94, admitted 16 April 1861.

43   Case Book IV, patient no. 231, admitted 12 November 1870.

44   Case Book II, patient no. 6, admitted 24 January 1863.

45   Case Book II, patient no. 172, admitted 27 April 1865.

46   Case Book II, patient no. 147, admitted 5 January 1865.

47   Case Book II, patient no. 143, admitted 17 December 1864.

48   Case Book II, patient no. 1, admitted 8 January 1863.

49   Case Book II, patient no. 12, admitted 23 March 1863.

50   Case Book II, patient no. 14, admitted 10 April 1863.

51   Case Book IV, patient no. 85, admitted 8 July 1869.

52   Case Book II, patient no. 139, admitted 17 November 1864.

53   *Asylums in Bengal for the Year 1877*, p. 33.

54   Minute by Pres.Madras, 29 October 1868, GOI (Public) Procs Feb 27 1869, 105–7A.

55   Chief Sec.Gvt.Madras to GOI, 26 November 1867, GOI (Public) Procs Feb 15 1868, 96A.

56   Off.Super.Bareilly.LA to IGP.NWP, 21 May 1868, GOI (Public) Procs Dec 19 1868, 49A.

57   *Asylums in the Central Provinces for the Year 1875*, p. 2.

58   M. Harrison, *Public Health in British India: Anglo-Indian preventive medicine 1859–1914* (Cambridge University Press Cambridge 1994), p. 19.

59   For nineteenth-century relationships between the body of the patient and the medical practitioner through the 'anatamo-clinical gaze' see M. Foucault, *The Birth of the Clinic: an archaeology of medical perception* (New York Vintage Books 1973), pp. 121–6; P. Major-Poetzl, *Michel Foucault's Archaeology of Western Culture: toward a new science of history* (Harvester Brighton 1983), pp. 144–6; D. Armstrong, 'Bodies of Knowledge/Knowledge of Bodies', in C. Jones and R. Porter (eds), *Reassessing Foucault: power, medicine and the body* (Routledge London 1994), pp. 17–27.

60   *Asylums in Bengal for the Year 1872*, p. 65.

61   Ibid., p. 65.

62   He is referring to John Thurnam, *Observations and Essays on the Statistics of Insanity* (London 1845).

63   *Asylums in Bengal for the Year 1870*, p. 7.

64   *Asylums in Bengal for the Year 1876*, p. 4.

65   *Asylums in Bengal for the Year 1873*, pp. 25–6.

66   *Asylums in the Madras Presidency during the Year 1878–9*, p. 12.

67   Author of, for example, *The Treatment of the Insane without Mechanical Restraints* (London 1856).

68   *Asylums in the Madras Presidency during the Year 1878–9*, p. 14.
69   *Asylums in the Madras Presidency during the Year 1877–78*, pp. 15–18.
70   Described as 'probably the outstanding philosopher-psychiatrist of the 19th century' by Henry Rollin, 'Whatever happened to Henry Maudsley?', in G. Berrios and H. Freeman (eds), *150 Years of British Psychiatry 1841– 1991* (Gaskell London 1991), p. 351.
71   Author of, for example, *Observations on the Structure of Hospitals for the Treatment of Lunatics as a Branch of Medical Police* (Edinburgh 1809).
72   Author of, for example, *The Borderlands of Insanity* (London 1875).
73   Author with Daniel Tuke of, for example, *A Manual of Psychological Medicine* (London 1874).
74   L. Ray, 'Models of Madness in Victorian asylum practice', in *Archives Européennes de Sociologie*, 22, 1981, p. 243.
75   Ibid., p. 241.
76   A. Scull, *Museums of Madness: the social organization of insanity in Nine-teenth-century England* (Penguin Middlesex 1982), p. 167.
77   Ibid., p. 167. This is a quote from Bucknill and Tuke, *A Manual of Psychological Medicine*.
78   *Asylums in the Central Provinces for the Year 1880*, p. 3.
79   A. Scull, *The Asylum as Utopia: W.A.F. Browne and the mid-nineteenth century consolidation of psychiatry* (Routledge London 1991), Introduc-tion, p. xxix.
80   *Indian Medical Gazette* review, viii, 1873, p. 135.
81   G. Berrios, 'Obsessional disorders during the nineteenth century: ter-minological and classificatory issues', in W. Bynum, R. Porter and M. Shepherd (eds), *The Anatomy of Madness: essays in the history of psy-chiatry* (Tavistock London 1985), p. 167.
82   G. Berrios, *The History of Mental Symptoms: descriptive psychopathology since the nineteenth-century* (Cambridge University Press Cambridge 1996), p. 21.
83   Ibid.
84   A. Scull, *The Asylum as Utopia*, Introduction p. xxiv.
85   Ibid., p. xxx.
86   Case Book IA, patient no. 15, admitted 13 May 1860.
87   Case Book IV, patient no. 20, admitted 14 December 1868.
88   Case Book IV, patient no. 22, admitted 30 December 1868.
89   Case Book IV, patient no. 36, admitted 20 February 1869.
90   For details see C. Bates, 'Racc, Caste and Tribe in Central India: the early origins of Indian anthropometry', in P. Robb (ed.), *The Concept of Race in South Asia* (Oxford University Press New Delhi 1995).
91   J. Urla and J. Terry, 'Introduction', in J. Urla and J. Terry (eds), *Devi-ant Bodies: critical perspectives on difference in science and popular culture* (Indiana University Press Bloomington), p. 1.
92   R. Tolen, 'Colonizing and Transforming the Criminal Tribesman: the Salvation Army in British India', in J. Urla and J. Terry (eds), *Deviant Bodies*, p. 81.
93   Case Book IA, patient no. 6, admitted 11 February 1860.
94   Case Book IV, patient no. 50, admitted 20 March 1869.
95   D. Arnold, *Colonizing the Body: state medicine and epidemic disease in nineteenth century India* (Oxford University Press New Delhi 1993), p. 8.

96 See J. Urla and J. Terry, 'Introduction', pp. 1–18.

97 Ibid., p. 4.

98 Case Book IA, patient no. 13, admitted 30 April 1860.

99 Y. Ripa, *Women and Madness: the incarceration of women in nineteenth-century France* (Polity Press Cambridge 1990), p. 160.

100 Ibid., p. 161.

101 E. Showalter, *The Female Malady: women, madness and English culture, 1830–1980* (Virago London 1987), p. 79.

102 J. Monk, 'Cleansing their Souls: laundries in institutions for fallen women', in *Lilith*, 9, 1996.

103 Case Book IV, patient no. 192, admitted 11 May 1870.

104 Case Book IA, patient no. 13, admitted 30 April 1860.

105 N. Rose, *The psychological complex: psychology, politics and society in England, 1869–1939* (Routledge London 1985), p. 45.

106 Ibid., p. 26.

107 M. MacMillan, 'Anglo-Indians and the Civilizing Mission 1880–1914', in G. Krishna (ed.), *Contributions to South Asian Studies 2* (Oxford University Press New Delhi 1982), p. 73.

108 L. Zastoupil, *John Stuart Mill and India* (Stanford University Press Stanford 1994), pp. 135–6.

109 N. Fraser, *Unruly Practices: power, discourse and gender in contemporary social theory* (Polity Press Cambridge 1989), p. 14.

110 See for example, S. Alatas, *The Myth of the Lazy Native: a study of the image of the Malays, Filipinos and Javanese from the 16th to the 20th century and its function in the ideology of colonial capitalism* (Frank Cass London 1977).

111 R. Inden, *Imagining India* (Basil Blackwell Oxford 1990), p. 264.

112 L. Zastoupil, *John Stuart Mill and India*, p. 175.

113 J. Majeed, *Ungoverned Imaginings: James Mill's 'History of British India' and Orientalism* (Clarendon Press Oxford 1992), p. 194.

114 E. Stokes, *The English Utilitarians and India* (Oxford University Press New Delhi 1959), p. 43.

115 Ibid., p. 56.

116 Case Book IA, patient no. 114, admitted 8 June 1861.

117 G. Risse and J. Warner, 'Reconstructing Clinical Activities', p. 189.

2 'The Lunatic Asylums of India are Filled with Ganja Smokers': Asylum Knowledge as Colonial Knowledge

1 D. Arnold, 'The Colonial Prison: power, knowledge and penology in nineteenth-century India', in D. Arnold and D. Hardiman (eds), *Subaltern Studies VIII* (Oxford University Press New Delhi 1994), p. 179.

2 'Papers relating to the consumption of ganja and other drugs in India', in *British Parliamentary Papers* (vol. 66 1893–4), p. 3.

3 Studies which examine attitudes towards opium and alcohol use in nineteenth century Britain include T. Parssinen and K. Kerner, 'Development of the disease model of drug addiction in Britain 1870–1926', in *Medical History*, 24, 1980; G. Harding, 'Constructing addiction as a moral failing',

in *Sociology of Health and Illness*, 8, 1986; B. Inglis, *The Forbidden Game: a social history of drugs* (Hodder and Stoughton London 1975); D. Peters, 'The British medical response to opiate addiction in the nineteenth century', in *Journal of the History of Medicine and Allied Sciences*, xxxvi, 1981.

4   'Papers relating to the consumption of ganja and other drugs in India', p. 7.

5   Ibid.

6   *Report of the Indian Hemp Drugs Commission 1893–4 (Mackworth-Young Commission)* (Government Printing Office Simla 1894), p. 1.

7   W. Ainslie, *Materia Indica* (London 1826), p. 109.

8   W. O'Shaughnessy, 'On the Preparations of the Indian Hemp, or Gunjah (Cannabis Indica): their effects on the animal system in health, and their utility in the treatment of tetanus and other convulsive diseases', in *Transactions of the Medical and Physical Society of Bengal*, 1838–1840. This paper was available in the Fitz-Hugh Ludlow Hypertext Library at website <http://www.nepenthes.com/Ludlow/> 1996. References are to page numbers of the text when downloaded and not to the original page numbers of 1838–40.

9   Ibid., p. 7.

10   Ibid., p. 14.

11   *The Enyclopaedia Britannica or Dictionary of Arts, Sciences and General Literature*, eighth edition 1856. This paper was available in the Fitz-Hugh Ludlow Hypertext Library at website <http://www.nepenthes.com/Ludlow/> 1998.

12   'Papers relating to the consumption of ganja and other drugs in India', pp. 7–8.

13   Ibid., p. 17.

14   Ibid., p. 29.

15   Ibid., p. 27.

16   Ibid., p. 35.

17   'Assaults by Ganja Smokers', in *Indian Medical Gazette*, xx, 1885, p. 220.

18   'Poisoning by Indian Hemp: Autopsy', in *The Lancet*, 10 April 1880, p. 585.

19   'Papers relating to the consumption of ganja and other drugs in India', p. 11.

20   Ibid., p. 65.

21   Ibid., p. 92.

22   Ibid., p. 78.

23   Ibid., p. 88.

24   A. Appadurai, 'Number in the Colonial Imagination', in C. Breckenridge and P. van der Veer (eds), *Orientalism and the Postcolonial Predicament: Perspectives on South Asia* (University of Pennsylvania Press Philadelphia 1993), p. 335.

25   Ibid., p. 319.

26   *Annual Report on the Insane Asylums in Bengal for the Year 1874*, p. 16.

27   Ibid.

28   For an investigation of certification processes in the UK see D. Wright, 'The Certification of Insanity in Nineteenth Century England and Wales', in *History of Psychiatry*, 9, 1998.

29 'Papers relating to the consumption of ganja and other drugs in India', p. 48.
30 S. Swartz, 'Colonizing the insane: causes of insanity in the Cape, 1891–1920', in *History of the Human Sciences*, 8, 1995, p. 40.
31 A. Scull, *The Asylum as Utopia: W.A.F. Browne and the mid-nineteenth century consolidation of psychiatry* (Routledge London 1991), Introduction, p. xxx.
32 Case Book IV, patient no. 38, admitted 23 February 1869.
33 Case Book II, patient no. 4, admitted 17 January 1863.
34 'Papers relating to the consumption of ganja and other drugs in India', pp. 14–15.
35 J. Goldstein, *Console and Classify: the French psychiatric profession in the nineteenth century* (Cambridge University Press Cambridge 1987), p. 378.
36 Ibid., p. 380.
37 D. de Giustino, *Conquest of Mind: Phrenology and Victorian Social Thought* (Croom Helm London 1975), p. 136.
38 Ibid., p. 139.
39 For a broader consideration of the importance of phrenology in colonial projects in India see C. Bates, 'Race, Caste and Tribe in Central India: the early origins of Indian anthropometry', in P. Robb (ed.), *The Concept of Race in South Asia* (Oxford University Press New Delhi 1995).
40 Case Book IA, patient no. 15, admitted 13 May 1860.
41 Case Book IV, patient no. 20, admitted 17 November 1868.
42 'Papers relating to the consumption of ganja and other drugs in India', p. 15.
43 *Asylums in Bengal for the Year 1868*, p. 37.
44 A. Appadurai, 'Number in the Colonial Imagination', p. 326.
45 *Asylums in Bengal for the Year 1867*, p. 10.
46 *Asylums in Bengal for the Year 1870*, p. 35.
47 *Asylums in Bengal for the Year 1875*, p. 24.
48 *Asylums in Bengal for the Year 1871*, p. 75.
49 *Asylums in Bengal for the Year 1872*, p. 65.
50 *Asylums in Bengal for the Year 1874*, p. 16.
51 *Asylums in the Punjab for the Year 1871–72*, p. 2.
52 *Report on the Lunatic Asylums in the Central Provinces for the Year 1880*, p. 7.
53 *Asylums in Bengal for the Year 1873*, p. 63.
54 Ibid., p. 3.
55 'Papers relating to the consumption of ganja and other drugs in India', p. 9.
56 Ibid., p. 12.
57 Ibid., p. 15.
58 Ibid., p. 88.
59 Ibid., p. 92.
60 *Report of the Indian Hemp Drugs Commission 1893–4*, p. 7.
61 Ibid., p. 231.
62 Ibid., p. 232.
63 Ibid.
64 Ibid., p. 236.

65   Ibid., p. 234.
66   Ibid., p. 225.
67   Ibid., p. 227.
68   Ibid.
69   Ibid.
70   Ibid.
71   Ibid., p. 237.
72   Ibid., p. 258.
73   'the *moderate* use of hemp drugs produces no injurious effects on the mind' [italics added] in ibid., p. 263.
74   B. Inglis, *The Forbidden Game*, p. 69.
75   See for example N. Rose who identifies the 'mapping of the population or at least its problematic sectors' as a process in modern government in 'Calculable minds and manageable individuals' in *History of the Human Sciences*, 1, 1988, p. 185.
76   *Asylums in Bengal for the Year 1867*, p. 73.
77   Case Book IA, patient no. 134, admitted 1 October 1861.

3   Disciplining Populations: British Admissions to 'Native-Only' Lunatic Asylums

1   Home (Public) December 19 1868, 46–59A.
2   Home (Public) December 19 1868, 51A.
3   'Annual Reports of the Lunatic Asylums at Bareilly and Benares for the year 1867', in *Selections from the Records of the Government of the North-Western Provinces*, p. 59.
4   W. Theobald, *The Legislative Acts of the Governor-General of India in Council* (Calcutta 1868).
5   *Annual Report of the Insane Asylums in Bengal for the Year 1862*, p. 34.
6   Case Book II, patient no. 151, admitted 7 February 1865.
7   Gvt.Ben. to GOI 21 July 1868 in Home (Public) 8 August 1868, 56–9A.
8   Case Book II, patient no. 7, admitted 12 February 1863.
9   Case Book II, patient no. 1, admitted 8 January 1863.
10   Case Book IA, patient no. 168, admitted 19 February 1862.
11   Case Book IV, patient no. 186, admitted 29 April 1870.
12   Case Book 1A, patient no. 124, admitted 2 August 1861.
13   Case Book IA, patient no. 139, admitted 4 October 1861.
14   *The Code of Criminal Procedure: An Act passed by the Legislative Council of India on the 5th September 1861* (London 1862): Section 295.
15   M. Radhakrishna, 'The Criminal Tribes Act in Madras Presidency: implications for itinerant trading communities', in *Indian Economic and Social History Review*, xxvi, 1989, p. 271.
16   *Report on the Administration of Criminal Justice in Oudh for the year 1880*, p. 7.
17   Ibid., p. 6.
18   Ibid.
19   Ibid.
20.   Case Book IA, patient no. 140, admitted 14 October 1861.

21 Case Book IA, patient not numbered (between 94 and 95), admitted 27 November 1861. This case note appears to have ended up out of sequence as the dates on 94 and 95 are for earlier in the year.

22 Oudh (General) 19 July 1876, 430B.

23 Oudh (General) 1 July 1874, 36B.

24 Order 3 February 1873 in Home (Public) June 1873, 78–9A.

25 R. Jütte, *Poverty and Deviance in Early Modern Europe* (Cambridge University Press Cambridge 1994), p. 147; G. Salgado, *The Elizabethan Underworld* (Dent London 1977), chapters 6, 7, 10; P. Slack, *Poverty and Policy in Tudor and Stuart England* (Longman London 1988), pp. 113–31; D. Garland, *Punishment and Welfare: a history of penal strategies* (Gower Aldershot 1985), p. 64.

26 N. Rose, *The Psychological Complex: psychology, politics and society in England 1869–1939* (Routledge London 1985), p. 45.

27 V. Oldenburg, *The Making of Colonial Lucknow 1856–1877* (Oxford University Press New Delhi 1989), pp. 18–64; A. King, *Colonial Urban Development: culture, social power and environment* (Routledge London 1976), p. 214.

28 Case Book II, patient no. 113, admitted 25 June 1864.

29 Case Book IV, patient no. 42, admitted 27 February 1869.

30 Case Book IV, patient no. 32, admitted 9 February 1869.

31 Case Book IA, patient no. 148, admitted 21 October 1861.

32 D. Hardiman (ed.), *Peasant Resistance in India 1858–1914* (Oxford University Press New Delhi 1993), p. 1.

33 T. Metcalf, *The Aftermath of Revolt: India 1857–1870* (Princeton University Press Princeton 1965), p. 305.

34 *Annual Report of the Lunatic Asylums of the Punjab for the year 1871–2*, p. 6.

35 T. Metcalf, *Ideologies of the Raj* (Cambridge University Press Cambridge 1994), p. 124.

36 On the segregation of Europeans in cantonments see A. King, *Colonial Urban Development*, pp. 97–122.

37 The development of racism as an ideology in British India has been described as a process where, 'the ideas forged in the crucible of 1857 were hammered into shape on the anvil of racial and political theory', in T. Metcalf, *The Aftermath of Revolt*, p. 310.

38 *Asylums in Bengal for the Year 1877*, p. 41.

39 *Asylums in Bengal for the Year 1879*, p. 19.

40 Statements attached to *Report on Dispensaries and Lunatic Asylums in the Province of Oudh for the Year 1875*.

41 *Report on the Lunatic Asylums in the Central Provinces for the Year 1876*, pp. 10–19; *Report on the Lunatic Asylums in the Central Provinces for the Year 1880*, pp. 12–14.

42 *Annual Administration and Progress Report on the Lunatic Asylums in the Bombay Presidency for the Year 1879*, pp. 8–10.

43 Statements attached to *Annual Report on the Lunatic Asylums in the Madras Presidency during the Year 1879–80*.

44 *Annual Report on the Jails of Bengal for the Year 1879*, p. xiii; *Report on the Jails of the Central Provinces for the Year 1879*, p. 4; *Report on the*

Condition and Management of Jails in the Province of Oudh for the Year 1875, p. 2; *Report on the Administration of the Jails of the Madras Presidency for the Year 1879*, p. 51; *Report on the Jails of the Punjab for the Year 1879*, p. 4; *Annual Report of the Bombay Jails for the Calendar Year 1879*, pp. 4–13.

45   J. Saunders, 'Magistrates and Madmen: segregating the criminally insane in late nineteenth-century Warwickshire' in V. Bailey (ed.), *Policing and Punishment in Nineteenth-Century Britain* (Croom Helm London 1981), pp. 221–2.

46   *Report on the administration of Criminal Justice in the Presidency of Bombay for the year 1879*, p. 31.

47   N. Walker and S. McCabe, *Crime and Insanity in England: new solutions and new problems, volume II* (Edinburgh University Press Edinburgh 1973), p. 50.

48   J. Eigen, *Witnessing Insanity: madness and mad-doctors in the English court* (Yale University Press London 1995), p. 106.

49   Ibid., p. 121.

50   This is explored in greater detail in Chapter 1.

51   This is explored in greater detail in Chapter 6.

52   'The labelling of the mad African as carried out in the colonial court room then, was often a confused and hesitant business', M. Vaughan, *Curing their Ills: colonial power and African illness* (Polity Press Cambridge 1991), p. 107.

53   NWP Judicial (Criminal) Proceedings July 1861, 89–91A: the account of this case is taken from the Session Judge's correspondence with the Government of the North-Western Provinces, 89–90A.

54   This is explored in greater detail in Chapter 2.

55   NWP Judicial (Criminal) Proceedings February 1861, 82–4A.

56   Deposition on Oath of the Civil Surgeon Saugar 13 December 1860, 83A.

57   R.B. Morgan's Opinion 8 January 1861, 83A.

58   For a consideration of the difficulties in using colonial legal records, see for example R. Guha, 'Chandra's Death' in R. Guha (ed.), *Subaltern Studies II* (Oxford University Press New Delhi 1983), or S. Amin, 'Approver's Testimony, Judicial Discourse: the case of Chauri Chaura' in R. Guha (ed.), *Subaltern Studies V* (Oxford University Press New Delhi 1987).

59   NWP Judicial (Criminal) January 1861, 32–4A.

60   Abstract of the Examination and Grounds and Date of Commitment for Trial 23 March 1860, 34A.

61   Civ.Asst.Surg. to Mag.Baitool 11 January 1860, 37A.

62   Civ.Asst.Surg. to Mag.Baitool 10 February 1860, 39A.

63   Deposition of Henry King 16 March 1860, 40A.

64   Gvt.NWP to Sessions Judge Saugar and Nerbudda 3 November 1860, 35A.

65   Translation of Evidence 8 November 1860, 40A.

66   Case Book IA, patient no. 10, admitted 14 March 1860.

67   Case Book IA, patient no. 156, admitted 14 December 1861.

68   J. Saunders, 'Magistrates and Madmen', pp. 225–6.

69 N. Walker and S. McCabe, *Crime and Insanity in England, volume II*, p. 38.
70 Ibid., p. 50.
71 S. Watson, 'Malingerers, the "weak-minded" criminal and the "moral imbecile": how the English prison medical officer became an expert in mental deficiency, 1880–1930', in M. Clark and C. Crawford (eds), *Legal Medicine in History* (Cambridge University Press Cambridge 1994), p. 234.
72 Ibid., p. 226.
73 Note on Jails and Jail Discipline in India 1867–68 by Arthur Howell in Home (Judicial) 9 January 1869, 39–52A.
74 Ibid.
75 This summary relies on details from the annual reports of the prisons mentioned which are summarised in Arthur Howell's Note.
76 Ibid.
77 Memorandum by Sir George Couper in Home (Judicial) 9 January 1869, 39–52A
78 'Punitive labour – one of the essential conditions of prison administration – appears often to have been made subsidiary to the introduction of remunerative forms of industry', from Gvt.Bengal to GOI in Home (Judicial) August 1875, 27–47A.
79 NWP Judicial (Criminal) 20 February 1864, 15–17B.
80 NWP Judicial (Criminal) 23 September 1865, 26B.
81 Home (Judicial) August 1875, 27–47A.
82 Gvt.C.Provs. to GOI 6 April 1875 in Ibid.
83 IGP.NWP to Gvt.NWP 22 March 1875 in Home (Judicial) August 1875, 27–47A.
84 IGP.NWP. to Gvt.NWP 11 December 1861 in Home (Judicial) 19 May 1862, 18–19A.
85 Resolution in Home (Judicial) 19 June 1869, 53–6A.
86 Oudh (General) 20 September 1872, 402B.
87 Case Book IA, patient no. 141, admitted 14 October 1861.
88 Case Book IA, patient no. 136, admitted 20 September 1861.
89 Case Book IA, patient no. 218, admitted 6 August 1862.
90 Case Book II, patient no. 184, admitted 29 May 1865.
91 Case Book IV, patient no. 216, admitted 20 August 1870.
92 Case Book IV, patient no. 101, admitted 17 August 1869.
93 See D. Arnold, 'The Colonial Prison: power, knowledge and penology in nineteenth-century India', in D. Arnold and D. Hardiman (eds), *Subaltern Studies VIII* (Oxford University Press New Delhi 1994), pp. 166–7.
94 Case Book IV, patient no. 101, admitted 17 August 1869.
95 Case Book IV, patient no. 156, admitted 2 February 1870.
96 V. Raghavan, *Law of Crimes: a single volume commentary on Indian Penal Code 1860 (Act no. 45 of 1860)* (Orient Law House New Delhi 1993).
97 Case Book II, patient no. 11, admitted 21 March 1863.
98 Case Book II, patient no. 124, admitted 8 August 1864.
99 Case Book II, patient no. 93, admitted 16 April 1864.
100 Case Book IV, patient no. 145, admitted 6 December 1869.

101   Case Book IA, patient no. 110, admitted 21 May 1861. Section 312 of the Indian Penal Code dealt with unlawful termination of pregnancies and stipulated that, 'A woman who causes herself to miscarry is within the meaning of this section.'

102   Case Book IA, patient no. 18, admitted 13 May 1860.

103   R. Smith, *Trial by Medicine: insanity and responsibility in Victorian trials* (Edinburgh University Press Edinburgh 1981), p. 144.

104   Ibid.

105   N. Walker, *Crime and Insanity in England, volume I*, p. 127.

106   Ibid., p. 128.

107   R. Smith, *Trial by Medicine*, p. 144.

108   R. Harris, *Murders and Madness: medicine, law and society in the fin de siècle* (Clarendon Press Oxford 1989), p. 35.

109   Ibid.

110   J. Wilson, *History of the Suppression of Infanticide in Western India under the Government of Bombay* (Smith and Taylor Bombay 1855), p. 430.

111   L. Panigrahi, *British Social Policy and Female Infanticide in India* (Munshiram Manoharlal New Delhi 1972), p. 121.

112   Ibid., p. 123.

113   It is interesting to note that when the Act was finally passed in 1870 the law member of the Government of India was Sir James Fitzjames Stephen, whose attitudes regarding insanity in cases where mothers murdered their children was mentioned earlier in this chapter and dealt with in N. Walker, *Crime and Insanity in England, volume I*.

114   L. Panigrahi, *British Social Policy and Female Infanticide*, p. 173.

115   Case Book IA, patient no. 76, admitted 10 January 1861.

116   W. Ernst, 'Idioms of Madness and Colonial Boundaries: the case of the European and "Native" mentally ill in early nineteenth-century British India', in *Society and History*, 39, 1997, p. 174.

4   Disciplining Individuals: Treatment Regimes Inside 'Native-Only' Lunatic Asylums

1   S. Sharma, *Mental Hospitals in India* (Directorate General of Health Services New Delhi 1990), p. 52.

2   Ibid., p. 53.

3   W. Ernst, *Mad Tales from the Raj: the European insane in British India 1800–1858* (Routledge London 1991), p. 166.

4   R. Paular, 'Mental Illness as a Social Problem in the Philippines during the Spanish Colonial Period', in *Philippine Journal of Psychology*, 25, 1992, p. 17: The author uses 'S' to stand for a *demente* (person who is mentally disturbed) admitted to the Hospicio de San Jose.

5   S. Swartz, 'The Black Insane in the Cape, 1891–1920', in *Journal of Southern African Studies*, 21, 1995, p. 411.

6   A. Scull, *Social Order/Mental Disorder: Anglo-American psychiatry in historical perspective* (Routledge London 1989), p. 89.

7   M. Foucault (translated by R. Howard), *Madness and Civilization: a history of insanity in the Age of Reason* (Routledge London 1989), p. 269.

8   Ibid., p. 266.
9   Y. Ripa, *Women and Madness: the incarceration of women in nineteenth-century France* (Polity Press Cambridge 1990), p. 123.
10 M. Finnane, *Insanity and the Insane in Post-Famine Ireland* (Croom Helm London 1981), p. 207.
11 Ibid., p. 205.
12 A. Digby, *Madness, Morality and Medicine: a study of the York Retreat, 1796–1914* (Cambridge University Press Cambridge 1985), pp. 128–9.
13 Ibid., p. 72.
14 M. Foucault, *Madness and Civilization*, p. 248.
15 D. Rothman, *The Discovery of the Asylum: social order and disorder in the New Republic* (Little Brown Boston 1971), p. 145.
16 Ibid., pp. 145–6.
17 E. Showalter, *The Female Malady: women, madness and English culture, 1830–1980* (Virago London 1987), p. 37.
18 Ibid., p. 82.
19 Y. Ripa, *Women and Madness*, p. 125.
20 M. Foucault, *Madness and Civilization*, p. 259.
21 'Annual Reports of the Lunatic Asylums at Bareilly and Benares for the Year 1866', in *Selections from the Records of the Government of the North-Western Provinces*, p. 61.
22 'Asylums at Bareilly and Benares for the Year 1867', p. 58.
23 D. Chakrabarty, 'The Difference-Deferral of a Colonial Modernity: public debates on domesticity in British Bengal', in D. Arnold and D. Hardiman (eds), *Subaltern Studies VIII* (Oxford University Press New Delhi 1994), p. 55.
24 Ibid.
25 *Annual Report on the Lunatic Asylums in the Punjab for the Year 1879*, p. 3.
26 Minute by President Madras 29 October 1865 GOI (Public) Procs, 27 February 1869, 105–7A.
27 *Asylums in the Punjab for the Year 1871–2*, p. 5.
28 *Annual Report of the Insane Asylums in Bengal for the Year 1863*, p. 3.
29 *Annual Administration and Progress Report on the Insane Asylums in the Bombay Presidency for the Year 1873–4*, p. 4.
30 *Asylums in Bengal for the Year 1867*, p. 93.
31 *Asylums in Bengal for the Year 1862*, p. 29.
32 *Asylums in the Punjab for the Year 1874*, p. 1.
33 *Asylums in the Bombay Presidency for the Year 1874–5*, p. 13.
34 *Asylums in the Bombay Presidency for the Year 1873–4*, p. 3: The decision to administer 'beef-tea' may have been taken as the patient in question was a Parsee rather than a Hindu. However it does seem to be an odd choice given the attitude of certain sections of the Indian community to vegetarian diets and cow products, so the decision to use the preparation may have reflected the ignorance of British medical officers about Indian diets or indeed may suggest something altogether more disciplinary. The superintendent may have had Eurocentric convictions about the benefits of meat in a diet and could have been attempting to force 'beef-tea' into the body against the will of the Indian patient in the belief that the Indian body must be

built and formed as the British wished it to be even if the Indian individual wanted to resist that form.

35   Ibid., p. 32.
36   *Asylums in Bengal for the Year 1862*, p. 66.
37   *Annual Report of the Three Lunatic Asylums in the Madras Presidency during the Year 1873–4*, p. 19.
38   D. Arnold, *Colonizing the Body: state medicine and epidemic disease in nineteenth century India* (Oxford University Press New Delhi 1993), p. 108.
39   *Asylums in the Madras Presidency during the Year 1873–4*, p. 22.
40   *Asylums in Bengal for the Year 1868*, p. 3.
41   *Asylums in Bombay for the Year 1876*, p. 9.
42   *Asylums in the Punjab for the Year 1871–2*, p. 3.
43   *Asylums in the Madras Presidency during the Year 1875–6*, p. 11.
44   *Asylums in Bengal for the Year 1862*, p. 66.
45   Civ.Surg.Rangoon to IMDBurma 15 January 1877, GOI (Medical) Procs October 1877, 18–20B.
46   Case Book IA, patient no. 114, admitted 8 June 1861.
47   Studies of colonial medicine and its impact on colonized bodies include R. Jeffery, *The Politics of Health in India* (University Of California London 1988); D. Arnold, 'Smallpox and colonial medicine in nineteenth century India', in D. Arnold (ed.), *Imperial Medicine and Indigenous Societies* (Oxford University Press New Delhi 1989); M. Harrison, *Public Health in British India: Anglo-Indian preventive medicine 1859–1914* (Cambridge University Press Cambridge 1994); R. Sheridan, *Doctors and Slaves: a medical and demographic history of slavery in the British West Indies 1680–1834* (Cambridge University Press Cambridge 1985); L. Stewart, 'The Edge of Utility: slaves and smallpox in the early eighteenth century', in *Medical History*, 29, 1985. For an especially vivid account of the disciplinary nature of the vaccination process see M. Vaughan, *Curing their Ills: colonial power and African illness* (Polity Press Cambridge 1991), p. 51.
48   *Asylums in the Madras Presidency during the Year 1877–8*, p. 12.
49   *Asylums at Bareilly and Benares for the Year 1867*, p. 58.
50   *Asylums in the Punjab for the Year 1871–2*, p. 1.
51   *Asylums in Bengal for the Year 1868*, p. 3.
52   Ibid.
53   *Asylums in the Bombay Presidency for the Year 1873–4*, p. 4.
54   *Asylums in the Punjab for the Year 1877*, p. 18.
55   *Asylums in the Madras Presidency during the Year 1877–8*, p. 6.
56   *Asylums in Bengal for the Year 1867*, p. 15.
57   Case Book IA, patient no. 175, admitted 6 March 1862.
58   Case Book IA, patient no. 56, admitted 24 September 1860.
59   A. Digby, *Madness, Morality and Medicine*, p. 128.
60   Comm.Rawul Pindee to Gvt.Punjab 2 January 1869, GOI (Judicial) 22 May 1869, 86A.
61   President Committee of Jail Enquiry to Gvt.Punjab 7 August 1869, GOI (Judicial) 9 October 1869, 27A.
62   Gvt.Punjab to GOI 17 August 1869, GOI (Judicial) October 9 1869, 26A.

63. Civ.Surg.Rawul Pindee to Asst.Comm.R.P. 21 July 1868, GOI (Judicial) 22 May 1869, 86A.
64. Civ.Surg.Rangoon to IMDBurma 15 January 1877, GOI (Medical) October 1877, 18–20B.
65. *Asylums in the Bombay Presidency for the Year 1873–4*, p. 3.
66. *Asylums in the Madras Presidency during the Year 1877–8*, p. 11.
67. *Asylums in the Madras Presidency during the Year 1876–7*, p. 22.
68. M. Foucault, *Madness and Civilization*, p. 266.
69. Case Book IA, patient no. 103, admitted 9 May 1861.
70. A seton was a strip of bandage sewn into the body to act as a counter irritant.
71. *Asylums in Bengal for the Year 1862*, p. 15.
72. *Asylums in the Bombay Presidency for the Year 1873–4*, p. 16.
73. Consider the paternalistic tone of Dr. Penny; 'Luxuries in the way of sweetmeats and fruit and the remains of public suppers have been constantly given in my own presence and by my own hands', in *Asylums in the Punjab for the Year 1870*, p. 3.
74 See for example, L. Zastoupil, *John Stuart Mill and India* (Stanford University Press Stanford 1994), p. 175; A. Nandy, *The Intimate Enemy: loss and recovery of self under colonialism* (Oxford University Press New Delhi), pp. 11–16.
75 A. Digby, 'Moral treatment at the Retreat 1796–1846', in W. Bynum, R. Porter and M. Shepherd (eds), *The Anatomy of Madness: essays in the history of psychiatry*, volume II (Tavistock London 1985), p. 68.
76. M. Foucault, *Madness and Civilization*, p. 252.
77. *Asylums in the Bombay Presidency for the Year 1874–5*, p. 28.
78. *Asylums in the Bombay Presidency for the Year 1873–4*, p. 16.
79. *Asylums in the Punjab for the Year 1876*, pp. 18–19.
80. *Asylums in Bengal for the Year 1862*, p. 66.
81. *Asylums in the Bombay Presidency for the Year 1873–4*, p. 44.
82. *Asylums in Bengal for the Year 1863*, p. 3.
83. *Asylums in Bengal for the Year 1862*, p. 72.
84. *Asylums in the Bombay Presidency for the Year 1873–4*, p. 29.
85. *Annual Inspection Report of the Dispensaries in Oudh for the Year 1872*, p. 299.
86. *Asylums in Bengal for the Year 1862*, p. 30.
87. *Asylums in the Bombay Presidency for the Year 1874–5*, p. 28.
88. *Asylums in the Bombay Presidency for the Year 1873–4*, p. 45.
89. *Asylums in the Punjab for the Year 1875*, p. 3.
90. R. Inden, *Imagining India* (Blackwell Oxford 1990), p. 133.
91. *Asylums in the Bombay Presidency for the Year 1873–4*, p. 30.
92. *Asylums in the Punjab for the Year 1874*, p. 2.
93. *Asylums in Bengal for the Year 1862*, p. 28.
94. *Asylums in the Bombay Presidency for the Year 1873–4*, p. 8.
95. Attachment in 'Reports on the Asylums for European and Native Insane Patients at Bhowanipore and Dullunda for 1856 and 1857', in *Selections from the Records of the Government of Bengal* no. XXVIII.
96. *Asylums in Bengal for the Year 1862*, p. 14.
97. *Asylums at Bareilly and Benares for the Year 1867*, p. 57.

98   *Asylums in the Bombay Presidency for the Year 1873–4*, p. 6.
99   *Asylums at Bareilly and Benares for the Year 1867*, pp. 57–58.
100 A. Appadurai, 'Number in the Colonial Imagination', in C. Breckenridge and P. van der Veer (eds), *Orientalism and the Postcolonial Predicament: perspectives on South Asia* (University of Pennsylvania Press Philadelphia 1993), p. 335.
101 *Asylums in Bengal for the Year 1862*, p. 15.
102 S. Sharma, *Mental Hospitals in India*, p. 52.
103 Ibid.
104 G. Chatterjee, *Child Criminals and the Raj* (Akshaya New Delhi 1995), p. 188.
105 L. Mathur, *Kala Pani: history of Andaman and Nicobar Islands with a study of India's Freedom Struggle* (Eastern Books Delhi 1985), p. 64.
106 P. Major-Poetzl, *Michel Foucault's Archaeology of Western Culture: toward a new science of history* (Harvester Brighton 1983), p. 204.
107 D. Arnold, 'The Colonial Prison: power, knowledge and penology in nineteenth-century India', in D. Arnold and D. Hardiman (eds), *Subaltern Studies VIII* (Oxford University Press New Delhi 1994), p. 187.
108 See for example S. Nigam, 'Disciplining and Policing the "Criminals by Birth", part 2: the development of a disciplinary system, 1871–1900', in *Indian Economic and Social History Review*, 27, 1990.
109 See for example R. Guha, 'Forestry and Social Protest in British Kumaun, c. 1893–91', in R. Guha (ed.), *Subaltern Studies IV* (Oxford University Press New Delhi 1985).
110 M. Vaughan, *Curing their Ills*, p. 11.
111 Ibid., p. 10.
112 *Report of the Lunatic Asylums at Bareilly and Benares for the Year 1867*, p. 59.
113 M. Foucault, *Discipline and Punish: the birth of the prison* (Penguin Harmondsworth 1979), p. 191.
114 M. Vaughan, *Curing their Ills*, p. 10.

5   Indians into Asylums: Local Communities and the Medical Institution

1   J. Paul, 'Medicine and Imperialism', in J. Ehrenreich (ed.), *The Cultural Crisis of Modern Medicine* (Monthly Review Press New York 1978), p. 282.
2   S. Sharma, *Mental Hospitals in India* (Directorate General of Health Services New Delhi 1990), p. 49.
3   S. Kakar, *Shamans, Mystics and Doctors: a psychological inquiry into India and its healing traditions* (Oxford University Press New Delhi 1982), p. 1.
4   M. Dols (edited by D. Immisch), *Majnun: the madman in medieval Islamic society* (Clarendon Oxford 1992).
5   S. Sharma, *Mental Hospitals in India*, p. 49.
6   S. Kakar, *Shamans, Mystics and Doctors*, pp. 60–5.
7   M. Foucault (translated by R. Howard), *Madness and Civilization: a history of insanity in the Age of Reason* (Routledge London 1989), p. 281.

8 Ibid., p. 257.
9 Ibid., p. 259.
10 S. Kakar, *Shamans, Mystics and Doctors*, p. 274.
11 N. Waxler, 'Is Mental Illness Cured in Traditional Societies? 'A theoretical analysis', in *Culture, Medicine and Psychiatry*, 1, 1977, p. 240.
12 Ibid.
13 S. Kakar, *Shamans, Mystics and Doctors*, p. 287.
14 N. Waxler, 'Is Mental Illness Cured in Traditional Societies?', p. 241.
15 S. Kakar, *Shamans, Mystics and Doctors*, p. 83.
16 P. Major-Poetzl, *Michel Foucault's Archaeology of Western Culture: toward a new science of history* (Harvester Brighton 1983), p. 132.
17 M. Foucault, *Madness and Civilization*, p. 269.
18 S. Sharma, *Mental Hospitals in India*, p. 49.
19 Case Book IA, patient no. 92, admitted 22nd March 1861.
20 R. Jeffery and P. Jeffery, 'A Woman Belongs to Her Husband', in A. Clark (ed.), *Gender and Political Economy: explorations of South Asian systems* (Oxford University Press New Delhi 1994), p. 94.
21 Bhagooie would not necessarily have to have acted oddly to have gained admission. 'Weak intellect' as a diagnosis seems to describe behaviour involving reluctance to speak or answer questions. Dullee (Case Book IA, patient no. 9, admitted 4 April 1860) is described as 'of weak intellect', and the only symptom noted is, 'very quiet, indeed never opens his mouth.' For Khooda Buksh (Case Book IA, patient no. 10, admitted 24 April 1860) the conclusion is that 'his intellect seems weak but he does not appear to labour under any delusion.' The behaviour noted on admission on which this is based is that he 'is very quiet and well-conducted'. It would seem then that had Bhagooie behaved as would be expected on her meeting with the European doctor, that is if she had displayed the reticence that would be natural for an Indian woman being addressed by a white, male official, she could have been diagnosed as of 'weak intellect', especially as the doctor had noted her dishevelled state on the basis of which he would have decided that her behaviour fitted into the familiar category of madness brought on by want. This was a link explicitly made in other cases, such as Madarow (Case Book II, patient no. 167, admitted 12 April 1865). The opinion is that 'this girl appears to have gone mad from starvation and bad treatment.'
22 Case Book IA, patient no. 97, admitted 20 April 1861.
23 The case note for Zahoorun (Case Book IA, patient no. 4, admitted 16 December 1859) is a good example of this. On admission her 'many hallucinations, such as the existence of a large snake in her belly', are remarked upon. Each entry thereafter makes reference to her beliefs. In December, three months after admission, a note is made that 'she fancies that she is possessed of great wealth and is the proprietress of hundreds of villages.' Three months later the entry observes that there is 'no alteration in her symptoms – the same fanciful notions about the snake + her imaginary wealth'. The next note adds that she thinks 'she is utterly starved in the asylum and is fed with dead men's flesh', and the final entry is that 'this woman continues to believe that she is fed with abominable filth. The snake left her 1000 years ago, that is to

say when she was 500 years old'. The fascination with the details of delusions is evident elsewhere. Whenever there is a lengthy note on Aluf (Case Book IV, patient no. 187, admitted 29 April 1870), his peculiarities are remarked upon. In 1870, 'hallucinations of a religious nature' are noted, in 1874, his remark, 'my eyes are burst from looking at the sun', and his statement that 'his penis is as big as his arm', are recorded and in 1878 the fact that he 'presents himself with a white flower stuck in each nostril', is put down. The delusions of Khooshal (Case Book II, patient no. 115, admitted 28 June 1864) are noted in each lengthy report on him after they come to light in 1868. 'Seems to have exalted ideas about his possessions. States that he has some lacs of horses and velvet harnesses', is followed up later with 'Is full of illusions as to immense wealth and possessions', and on other occasions his comments that 'I have 9 lacs of elephants' and 'Formerly I used to eat gold and silver', are recorded.

24 The reasons for seeking transfer from prison to asylum are discussed in greater detail in Chapter 3.
25 Case Book II, patient no. 130, admitted 30 August 1864.
26 *Report on the Lunatic Asylums in the Central Provinces for the Year 1879*, p. 1.
27 Case Book IA, patient no. 193, admitted 5 May 1862.
28 *Indian Medical Gazette*, Vol. XII, March 1 1877, p. 76.
29 Case Book II, patient no. 222, admitted 28 September 1865.
30 Case Book IA, patient no. 128, admitted 24th August 1861.
31 Case Book II, patient no. 158, admitted 28th February 1865: case note transcribed as on original.
32 Deposition of Seetul Sonar in NWP Judicial (Criminal) March 1864, 14A.
33 Super.Police Goruckpore to I.G.Police Benares 22 October 1863 in NWP Judicial (Criminal) March 1864, 26A.
34 M. Finnane, *Insanity and the Insane in post-Famine Ireland* (Croom Helm London 1981), p. 163.
35 Ibid. For the importance of the family in asylum admissions see also M. Finnane, 'Asylums, Families and the State', in *History Workshop Journal*, 20, 1985; P. Bartlett, *The Poor Law of Lunacy: the administration of pauper lunatics in mid-nineteenth century England, with special emphasis on Leicestershire and Rutland* (unpublished thesis University College London 1993); D. Wright, 'Getting Out of the Asylum: understanding the confinement of the insane in the nineteenth century', in *Social History of Medicine*, 10, 1997. Wright goes as far as to argue that in the UK in the nineteenth century 'although small numbers of inmates may indeed have been arrested and confined for vagrancy, the majority were admitted to asylums by family members', p. 145. This is certainly not the case in India in the period of this study.
36 Case Book II, patient no. 149, admitted 1 February 1865.
37 Case Book IA, patient no. 202, admitted 10 June 1862.
38 Case Book II, patient no. 70, admitted 8 December 1863.
39 E. Showalter, *The Female Malady: women, madness and English culture, 1830–1980* (Virago London 1987), p. 58.

40 A village midwife quoted in R. Jeffery and P. Jeffery, 'A Woman Belongs to Her Husband', p. 99.

41 Ibid., p. 100.

42 Case Book IV, patient no. 202, admitted 15 June 1870.

43 For example, Hanooman's notes (Case Book IA, patient no. 222, admitted 20 August 1862) record that he 'had previously been an inmate in the Asylum and was discharged in July 1861'. The tracing of previous admissions seems to have been so efficient that those treated in the Jail Hospital for insanity before the establishment of the Asylum have it noted when admitted into the Asylum. Kurreem Buy (Case Book IA, patient no. 40, admitted 20 July 1860) was 'once in the Asylum in the Jail'.

44 For example, another puerperal maniac is admitted 3 months after Mosst. Goolaba. Mosst.Rhuman (Case Book IV, patient no. 220, admitted 15 September 1870) was 'Certified by the Magistrate Violent'. She was handed over to her husband 8 months later.

45 Case Book II, patient no. 3, admitted 15 January 1863.

46 N. Waxler, 'Is Mental Illness Cured in Traditional Societies?', p. 239.

47 Ibid., p. 243.

48 Ibid., p. 248.

49 Case Book II, patient no. 38, admitted 16 June 1863.

50 M. Harrison, *Public Health in British India: Anglo-Indian preventive medicine 1859–1914* (Cambridge University Press Cambridge 1994), p. 232.

51 D. Arnold, 'Smallpox and colonial medicine in nineteenth century India', in D. Arnold (ed.), *Imperial Medicine and Indigenous Societies* (Oxford University Press New Delhi 1988), p. 62.

52 D. Arnold, *Colonizing the Body: state medicine and epidemic disease in nineteenth-century India* (Oxford University Press New Delhi 1993), p. 250.

53 Ibid., p. 248.

54 M. Harrison, *Public Health in British India*, p. 89.

55 D. Arnold, *Colonizing the Body*, p. 250

56 The multitude of duties that the Civil Surgeon was required to attend to is discussed further in a focus on the staffing arrangements of the asylums in Chapter VI.

57 For dispensary finance see M. Harrison, *Public Health in British India*, p. 88: for asylum finances see the Conclusion.

58 *Report on the Asylums, Vaccination and Dispensaries in Bengal, 1868–1873*, p. 13.

6 Indians inside Asylums: Staff, Patients and Power

1. Case Book IV, patient no. 42, admitted 27 February 1869.

2. A. Beveridge, 'Life in the Asylum: patients' letters from Morningside, 1873–1908', in *History of Psychiatry*, 9, 1998, p. 461.

3. Z. Pathak and R. Rajan, 'Shahbano', in *Signs*, 14, 1989, p. 572.

4. S. Ortner, 'Resistance and the Problem of Ethnographic Refusal', in *Comparative Study of Society and History*, 37, 1995, p. 185.

5. M. Foucault (translated by R. Howard), *Madness and Civilization: a history of insanity in the age of reason* (Routledge London 1989), p. 262.

6   Case Book IV, patient no. 42, admitted 27 February 1869.
7   N. Dirks, G. Eley and S. Ortner (eds), *Culture/Power/History: a reader in contemporary social theory* (Princeton University Press Princeton 1994), p. 19.
8   C. Quétel (translated by J. Braddock and B. Pike), *History of Syphilis* (Polity Press 1990), p. 160.
9   J. Walton (ed.), *Brain's Diseases of the Nervous System 10th Edition* (Oxford University Press Oxford 1993), p. 291.
10 J. Wise, 'General Paralysis of the Insane', in *Indian Medical Gazette*, iv, 1869, p. 76.
11 Ibid., p. 76.
12 N. Dirks *et al.*, *Culture/Power/History*, p. 18.
13 R. Russell, 'The lunacy profession and its staff in the second half of the nineteenth century, with special reference to the West Riding Lunatic Asylum', in W. Bynum, R. Porter and M. Shepherd (eds), *The Anatomy of Madness: essays in the history of psychiatry volume III* (Routledge London 1988), p. 312; see also L. Monk, 'Working like Mad: nineteenth century female lunatic asylum attendants and violence', in *Lilith*, 9, 1996.
14 R. Russell, 'The lunacy profession and its staff', p. 312.
15 H. Deacon, *A History of the Medical Institutions on Robben Island, Cape Colony, 1846–1910* (Cambridge unpublished thesis 1994), pp. 100–1.
16 W. Ernst, *Mad Tales from the Raj: the European insane in British India, 1800–1858* (Routledge 1991), p. 106.
17 D. Arnold, *Colonizing the Body: state medicine and epidemic disease in nineteenth-century India* (Oxford University Press New Delhi 1993), p. 6.
18 M. Lyons, 'The Power to Heal: African medical auxiliaries in colonial Belgian Congo and Uganda', in D. Engels and S. Marks (eds), *Contesting Colonial hegemony: state and society in Africa and India* (British Academic Press 1994), p. 222.
19 *Annual Report of the Insane Asylums in Bengal for the Year 1880*, p. 36.
20 *Annual Report of the Lunatic Asylums of the Punjab for the Year 1880*, p. 12.
21 J. Thornton, *Memories of Seven Campaigns: a record of thirty-five years' service in the Indian Medical Department in India, China, Egypt and the Sudan* (London 1895), pp. 168–72.
22 *Asylums in Bengal for the Year 1878*, p. 23.
23 Ibid., p. 27.
24 *Annual Inspection Report of the Dispensaries in Oudh for the Year 1872*, p. 28.
25 *Asylums in Bengal for the Year 1869*, p. 4.
26 *Asylums in Bengal for the Year 1869*, p. 5.
27 *Asylums in Bengal for the Year 1876*, p. 35.
28 *Asylums in the Punjab for the Year 1876*, p. 19.
29 Extract of letter from IGP British Burma 28 September 1870 in GOI (Public) Procs 8 April 1871, 38–9A.
30 R. O'Hanlon, 'Recovering the Subject: Subaltern Studies and histories of resistance in colonial South Asia', in *Modern Asian Studies* 22, 1988, p. 214.
31 *Asylums in Bengal for the Year 1877*, p. 134.

32 *Asylums in Bengal for the Year 1878*, p. 23.
33 *Asylums in the Punjab for the Year 1874*, p. 12.
34 *Asylums in Bengal for the Year 1869*, pp. 4–5.
35 *Asylums in Bengal for the Year 1870*, p. 18.
36 'Reports on the Asylums for European and Native Insane Patients at Bhowanipore and Dullunda for 1856 and 1857', in *Selections from the Records of the Government of India* no. XXVIII, p. 63.
37 'Annual Reports of the Lunatic Asylums at Bareilly and Benares for the Year 1867', in *Selections from the Records of the Government of the North-Western Provinces*, p. 59.
38 *Annual Report of the Three Lunatic Asylums in the Madras Presidency during the Year 1873–4*, p. 13.
39 *Asylums in the Madras Presidency during the Year 1877–8*, p. 25.
40 'Asylums at Bareilly and Benares for the Year 1867', p. 47.
41 *Asylums in Bengal for the Year 1878*, p. 7.
42 *Asylums in Bengal for the Year 1870*, p. 12.
43 *Asylums in the Punjab for the Year 1876*, p. 11.
44 *Asylums in the Punjab for the Year 1870*, p. 15.
45 *Asylums in the Punjab for the Year 1871–2*, p. 5.
46 *Asylums in the Punjab for the Year 1875*, p. 3.
47 *Asylums in Bengal for the Year 1877*, p. 29.
48 This is discussed in greater detail in Chapter 4.
49 *Asylums in Bengal for the Year 1877*, p. 27.
50 *Asylums in Bengal for the Year 1878*, p. 24.
51 Ibid., p. 15.
52 *Dispensaries in Oudh for the Year 1869*, p. 2.
53 *Dispensaries in Oudh for the Year 1873*, p. 3.
54 *Asylums in Bengal for the Year 1869*, p. 7.
55 Gvt.Oudh to GOI 12 August 1868 3403, in GOI (Public) Procs December 19 1868, 25A.
56 *Asylums in Bengal for the Year 1880*, p. 37
57 Ibid; Cuttack produced goods sold off for Rs 1223 in 1880 with an average asylum population of just 51 patients.
58 *Asylums in the Punjab for the Year 1880*, p. 3.
59 *Asylums at Bareilly and Benares for the Year 1866*, p. 33.
60 M. Lyons, 'The Power to Heal', pp. 219–22.
61 *Asylums in Bengal for the Year 1863*, p. 3.
62 *Asylums in the Bombay Presidency for the Year 1873–4*, p. 44.
63 *Asylums in Bengal for the Year 1862*, p. 31.
64 Case Book IA, patient no. 142, admitted 14 October 1861: underlining in original.
65 Case Book IA, patient no. 210, admitted 24 July 1862.
66 See for example, S. Alatas, *The Myth of the Lazy Native: a study of the image of the Malays, Filipinos and Javanese from the 16th to the 20th century and its function in the ideology of colonial capitalism* (Frank Cass London 1977).
67 *Asylums in Bengal for the Year 1863*, p. 29.
68 *Asylums in Bengal for the Year 1862*, p. 14.
69 *Asylums in the Central Provinces for the Year 1877*, p. 1.

70   *Asylums in the Madras Presidency during the Year 1877–8*, p. 14.
71   *Asylums in the Madras Presidency during the Year 1878–9*, p. 14.
72   *Asylums in the Bombay Presidency for the Year 1876*, p. 18.
73   *Asylums in the Central Provinces for the Year 1879*, p. 2.
74   Case Book IA, patient no. 75, admitted 7 January 1861.
75   *Asylums in the Central Provinces for the Year 1880*, p. 2.
76   *Asylums in Bengal for the Year 1878*, p. 7.
77   IGH Lower Provinces to Gvt.Bengal 27 July 1868 288, in GOI (Public) Procs December 19 1868, 30A.
78   It is safe to assume that the staff member was Indian as European staff exclusively occupy the posts of Deputy Superintendent, Overseer or Matron in the records.
79   See A. Skaria, 'Writing, Orality and Power in the Dangs, Western India, 1800s–1920' in *Subaltern Studies IX* (Oxford University Press New Delhi 1997).
80   *Annual Report of the Lahore Lunatic Asylum for the Year 1868*, p. 4.
81   *Asylums in the Bombay Presidency for the Year 1873–4*, p. 3.
82   Gvt.C.Provs to Dr. Beatson 23 February 1875, 675–31 in GOI (Medical) Procs November 1875, 16A.
83   This is discussed in greater detail in Chapter 4.
84   Dr. Beatson to Gvt.C.Provs 23 February 1875, 12 in GOI (Medical) Procs November 1875, 20A.
85   Minute by W.B. Jones 25 October 1873 in GOI (Medical) Procs November 1875, 16A.
86   Dr. Beatson to Gvt.C.Provs 23 February 1875, 12 in GOI (Medical) Procs November 1875, 20A.
87   *Asylums in the Bombay Presidency for the Year 1877*, p. 52.
88   Ibid., p. 11.
89   *Asylums in the Bombay Presidency for the Year 1876*, p. 26.
90   *Asylums in Bengal for the Year 1873*, p. 38.
91   Case Book IA, patient no. 2, admitted 14 November 1859.
92   Case Book IA, patient no. 81, admitted 1 February 1861.
93   *Lahore Lunatic Asylum for the Year 1868*, p. 4.
94   *Asylums in Bengal for the Year 1863*, p. 29.
95   *Asylums in the Bombay Presidency for the Year 1876*, p. 26.
96   Case Book IA, patient no. 152, admitted 21 November 1861.
97   S. Ortner, 'Resistance and the Problem of Ethnographic Refusal', in *Comparative Study of Society and History* 1995, p. 175.
98   R. O'Hanlon, 'Recovering the Subject', p. 223.
99   J. Scott, *Weapons of the Weak: everyday forms of peasant resistance* (Yale University Press New Haven 1985), p. 297.

Conclusion

1   A. Camus (translated by S. Gilbert), *The Plague* (Penguin 1960), p. 250.
2   Gvt.NWP to GOI 2155A of 1862 in GOI (Public) 20 October 1862, 26A.
3   IGP to Gvt.NWP 30 June 1862 in GOI (Public) 20 October 1862, 27A.
4   *Report on the Lunatic Asylums in Bengal by the Committee appointed to inquire into medical expenditure in Bengal.*

5 G. Risse and J. Warner, 'Reconstructing Clinical Activities: patient records and medical history', in *Social History of Medicine*, 5, 1992, p. 189.

6 D. Arnold, *Colonizing the Body: state medicine and epidemic disease in nineteenth-century India* (Oxford University Press New Delhi 1993).

7 Super. Police Pahlunpore to Gvt.Bombay 15 February 1868 in GOI (Judicial) 19 February 1870, 21–35A.

8 Officer Southern District to Officer Northern District 21 January 1879 in GOI (Port Blair) May 1879, 42–3B: the 'asylum' at Haddo was in fact no such thing as understood by the standards of the day. Correspondence in 1876 (Home [Port Blair] November 1876, 4–7A) established that there was simply a separate shed at Haddo in which all the convicts 'who will submit to no discipline' were sent to separate them out from the other prisoners.

9 N. Dirks, 'Introduction: Colonialism and Culture' in N. Dirks (ed.), *Colonialism and Culture* (Ann Arbor Michigan 1992), p. 23.

10 M. Foucault (translated by R. Howard), *Madness and Civilization: a history of insanity in the age of reason* (Routledge London 1989), pp. 257–9.

11 N. Thomas, *Colonialism's Culture: anthropology, travel and government* (Polity Press Cambridge 1994), p. 57.

12 W. Keane, 'From Fetishism to Sincerity: on agency, the speaking subject and their historicity in the context of religious conversion', in *Comparative Study of Society and History*, 39, 1997, p. 674.

13 N. Dirks, G. Eley and S. Ortner (eds), *Culture/Power/History: a reader in contemporary social theory* (Princeton University Press Princeton 1994), p. 18.

14 R. O'Hanlon, 'Recovering the Subject: Subaltern Studies and histories of resistance in colonial South Asia', in *Modern Asian Studies* 22, 1988, p. 191.

15 Ibid., p. 216.

Bibliography

Unpublished Sources

Agra Mental Hospital

Lucknow Lunatic Asylum Case Notes (1859–1872).

Edinburgh University Medical Archive

Robertson Milne-Collection.

India Office Library

Bengal Military Proceedings.
Military Letters received from Bengal.

National Archives of India

GOI Home (Judicial) Proceedings.
GOI Home (Medical) Proceedings.
GOI Home (Port Blair) Proceedings.
GOI Home (Public) Proceedings.

UP State Archive (Lucknow)

North-Western Provinces Judicial (Criminal) Proceedings.
Oudh (General) Proceedings.

Published Official Sources

India Office Library

Report of the Indian Hemp Drugs Commission 1893–4 (Mackworth-Young Commission), (Simla 1894).

Asylums

Selections from the Records of the Government of Bengal (Calcutta 1859).
Annual Reports on the Insane Asylums in Bengal (Calcutta 1862–1880).
Report on the Lunatic Asylums in Bengal by the Committee appointed to inquire into medical expenditure in Bengal (Calcutta 1879).
General Report no. 6 on the Lunatic Asylums, Vaccination and Dispensaries in the Bengal Presidency 1873 (Calcutta 1876).
Annual Administration and Progress Reports on the Insane Asylums in the Bombay Presidency (Bombay 1873–1880).
Reports on the Lunatic Asylums in the Central Provinces (Nagpur 1869–1880).
Annual Reports on the Lunatic Asylums in the Madras Presidency (Madras 1874–1880).
Selections from the Records of the Government of the North-Western Provinces (Allahabad 1868).
Annual Inspection Reports of the Dispensaries in Oudh (Lucknow 1868–1875).
Annual Reports of the Lunatic Asylums of the Punjab (Lahore 1867–1880).

Jails

Annual Report on the Jails of Bengal for the Year 1879 (Calcutta 1880).
Annual Report of the Bombay Jails for the Calendar Year 1879 (Bombay 1880).
Report on the Jails of the Central Provinces for the Year 1879 (Nagpur 1880).
Report on the Administration of the Jails of the Madras Presidency for the Year 1879 (Madras 1880).
Report on the Condition and Management of Jails in the Province of Oudh for the Year 1875 (Lucknow 1876).
Report on the Jails of the Punjab for the Year 1879 (Lahore 1880).

Justice

The Code of Criminal Procedure: An Act passed by the Legislative Council of India on the 5th September 1861 (London 1862).
Report on the Administration of Criminal Justice in Oudh for the Year 1880 (Lucknow 1881).
Report on the Administration of Criminal Justice in the Presidency of Bombay for the Year 1879 (Bombay 1880).

Edinburgh University Library

British Parliamentary Papers: 'Papers relating to the consumption of ganja and other drugs in India' (Vol. 66 1893–4).

Published Primary Sources

Indian Medical Gazette.
Encyclopædia Britannica or dictionary of arts, sciences, and general literature (eighth edition, Boston, MDCCLVI).
Lancet.
Transactions of the Medical and Physical Society of Bengal.
Ainslie, W. *Materia Indica* (London 1826).

Bucknill, J.C. and Tuke, D. *A Manual of Psychological Medicine* (London 1874).
Duncan, A. *Observations on the Structure of Hospitals for the Treatment of Lunatics as a Branch of Medical Police* (Edinburgh 1809).
Dunglison, R. *New Remedies, Pharmaceutically and Therapeutically Considered* (Philadelphia 1843).
Johnston, J.F. *Chemistry of Common Life* (New York 1855).
Mill, J. *The History of British India*, Vol. II (London 1858).
Theobald, W. *The Legislative Acts of the Governor-General of India in Council* (Calcutta 1868).
Thornton, J.H. *Memories of Seven Campaigns: a record of thirty-five years' service in the Indian Medical Department in India, China, Egypt and the Sudan* (London 1895).
Thurnam, J. *Observations and Essays on the Statistics of Insanity* (London 1845).
Wilson, J. *History of the Suppression of Infanticide in Western India under the Government of Bombay* (Bombay 1855).
Wise, J. 'General Paralysis of the Insane', in *Indian Medical Gazette*, iv, 1869.
Wynter, A. *The Borderlands of Insanity* (London 1875).

Published and Unpublished Secondary Sources

Alatas, S. *The Myth of the Lazy Native: a study of the image of the Malays, Filipinos and Javanese from the 16th to the 20th century and its function in the ideology of colonial capitalism* (Frank Cass London 1977).
Albarn, T. 'Age and Empire in the Indian Census, 1871–1931', in *Journal of Interdisciplinary History*, xxx, 1999.
Amin, S. 'Approver's Testimony, Judicial Discourse: the case of Chauri Chaura' in R. Guha (ed.), *Subaltern Studies V* (Oxford University Press New Delhi 1987).
Andrews, J. 'Case Notes, Case Histories, and the Patient's Experience of Insanity at Gartnavel Royal Asylum, Glasgow, in the Nineteenth Century', in *Social History of Medicine*, 11, 1998.
Appadurai, A. 'Number in the Colonial Imagination', in C. Breckenridge and P. van der Veer (eds), *Orientalism and the Postcolonial Predicament: perspectives on South Asia* (University of Pennsylvania Press Philadelphia 1993).
Armstrong, D. 'Bodies of Knowledge/Knowledge of Bodies', in C. Jones and R. Porter (eds), *Reassessing Foucault: power, medicine and the body* (Routledge London 1994).
Arnold, D. *Police Power and Colonial Rule: Madras 1859–1947* (Oxford University Press New Delhi 1986).
Arnold, D. *Imperial Medicine and Indigenous Societies* (Oxford University Press New Delhi 1988).
Arnold, D. *Colonizing the Body: state medicine and epidemic disease in nineteenth-century India* (Oxford University Press New Delhi 1993).
Arnold, D. 'The Colonial Prison: power, knowledge and penology in nineteenth-century India', in D. Arnold and D. Hardiman (eds), *Subaltern Studies VIII: essays in honour of Ranajit Guha* (Oxford University Press New Delhi 1994).
Bartlett, P. *The Poor Law of Lunacy: the administration of pauper lunatics in*

mid-nineteenth century England, with special emphasis on Leicestershire and Rutland (unpublished thesis University College London 1993)

Bates, C. 'Race, caste and tribe in central India: the early origins of Indian anthropometry', in P. Robb (ed.), *The Concept of Race in South Asia* (Oxford University Press New Delhi 1995).

Berridge, V. and Edwards, G. *Opium and the People: opiate use in nineteenth century England* (St. Martin's Press London 1981).

Berrios, G. 'Obsessional disorders during the nineteenth century: terminological and classificatory issues', in W. Bynum, R. Porter and M. Shepherd (eds), *The Anatomy of Madness: essays in the history of psychiatry* (Tavistock London 1985).

Berrios, G. *The History of Mental Symptoms: descriptive psychopathology since the nineteenth-century* (Cambridge University Press Cambridge 1996).

Beveridge, A. 'Madness in Victorian Edinburgh: a study of patients admitted to the Royal Edinburgh Asylum under Thomas Clouston 1873–1908', Part I in *History of Psychiatry*, 6, 1995; Part II in *History of Psychiatry*, 6, 1995.

Beveridge, A. 'Life in the Asylum: patients' letters from Morningside, 1873–1908', in *History of Psychiatry*, 9, 1998.

Castel, R. *The Regulation of Madness: the origins of incarceration in France* (Polity Press Oxford 1988).

Chakrabarty, D. 'The Difference-Deferral of a Colonial Modernity: public debates on domesticity in British Bengal', in D. Arnold and D. Hardiman (eds), *Subaltern Studies VIII* (Oxford University Press New Delhi 1994).

Chatterjee, G. *Child Criminals and the Raj: reformation in British jails* (Akshaya New Delhi 1995).

Chesler, P. *Women and Madness* (Allen Lane London 1984).

Cohn, B. 'The Census, Social Structure and Objectification in South India', in B. Cohn (ed.), *An Anthropologist among the Historians and Other Essays* (Oxford University Press New Delhi 1987).

Coleborne, C. 'Legislating lunacy and the body of the female lunatic', in D. Kirkby (ed.), *Sex, Power and Justice: historical perspectives on law in Australia* (Oxford University Press Melbourne 1995).

Coleborne, C. 'Gender and the Patient case-book in the lunatic asylum in colonial Victoria (Australia)', presented to the Society for the Social History of Medicine *Medicine and the Colonies Conference*, Oxford 1996.

Coleborne, C. '"She does her hair up fantastically": the production of femininity in patient case books of the lunatic asylum in 1860s Victoria', in J. Long (ed.), *Forging Identities: bodies, gender and feminist history* (University of Western Australia Press Nedlands 1997).

Deacon, H. *A History of the Medical Institutions on Robben Island, Cape Colony 1846–1910* (unpublished thesis Cambridge 1994).

de Giustino, D. *Conquest of Mind: phrenology and Victorian social thought* (Croom Helm London 1975).

Digby, A. *Madness, Morality and Medicine. A study of the York Retreat 1796–1914* (Cambridge University Press Cambridge 1985).

Digby, A. 'Moral treatment at the Retreat 1796–1846', in W. Bynum, R. Porter and M. Shepherd (eds), *The Anatomy of Madness: essays in the history of psychiatry*, volume II (Tavistock London 1985).

Dirks, N. *Colonialism and Culture* (Ann Arbor Michigan 1992).

Dirks, N. Eley, G. and Ortner, S. *Culture/Power/History: a reader in contemporary social theory* (Princeton University Press Princeton 1994).

Dols, M. (edited by D. Immisch), *Majnun: the madman in medieval Islamic society* (Clarendon Oxford 1992).

Dwyer, E. *Homes for the Mad: life inside two nineteenth-century asylums* (Rutgers University Press New Brunswick 1987)

Eigen, J. *Witnessing Insanity: madness and mad-doctors in the English court* (Yale University Press London 1995).

Ernst, W. *Mad Tales from the Raj: the European insane in British India 1800–1858* (Routledge London 1991).

Ernst, W. 'Idioms of Madness and Colonial Boundaries: the case of the European and "Native" mentally ill in early nineteenth-century British India', in *Comparative Study in Society and History*, 39, 1997.

Fairclough, N. *Critical Discourse Analysis: the critical study of language* (Longman London 1995)

Fanon, F. 'Medicine and Colonialism', in J. Ehrenreich (ed.), *The Cultural Crisis of Modern Medicine* (Monthly Review Press New York 1978).

Finnane, M. *Insanity and the Insane in Post-Famine Ireland* (Croom Helm London 1981).

Finnane, M. 'Asylums, Families and the State', in *History Workshop Journal*, 20, 1985.

Foucault, M. *The Birth of the Clinic: an archaeology of medical perception* (Vintage Books New York 1973).

Foucault, M. (translated by Richard Howard), *Madness and Civilization: a history of insanity in the Age of Reason* (Routledge London 1989).

Fraser, N. *Unruly Practices: power, discourse and gender in contemporary social theory* (Polity Press Cambridge 1989)

Garland, D. *Punishment and Welfare: a history of penal strategies* (Gower Aldershot 1985).

Garton, S. *Medicine and Madness: a social history of insanity in New South Wales, 1880–1940* (New South Wales University Press Kensington NSW 1988).

Goldstein, J. *Console and Classify: the French psychiatric profession in the nineteenth century* (Cambridge University Press Cambridge 1987).

Grob, G. *Mental Institutions in America: social policy to 1875* (NY Free Press New York 1973)

Guha, R. 'On Some Aspects of the Historiography of Colonial India', in R. Guha (ed.), *Subaltern Studies I* (Oxford University Press New Delhi 1982).

Guha, R. 'The Prose of Counter-Insurgency', in R. Guha, *Subaltern Studies II* (Oxford University Press New Delhi 1983).

Guha, R. 'Forestry and Social Protest in British Kumaun, c. 1893–91', in R. Guha (ed.), *Subaltern Studies IV* (Oxford University Press New Delhi 1985).

Guha, R. 'Chandra's Death', in R. Guha (ed.), *Subaltern Studies V* (Oxford University Press New Delhi 1987).

Hacking, I. 'Making Up People', in T. Heller, M. Sosna and D. Wellerby (eds), *Reconstructing Individualism: autonomy, individuality and the self in Western thought* (Stanford University Press Stanford 1986).

Hardiman, D. (ed.), *Peasant Resistance in India 1858–1914* (Oxford University Press New Delhi 1993).

Harding, G. 'Constructing addiction as a moral failing', in *Sociology of Health and Illness*, 8, 1986.

Harris, R. *Murders and Madness: medicine, law and society in the fin de siècle* (Clarendon Press Oxford 1989).

Harrison, M. *Public Health in British India: Anglo-Indian preventive medicine 1859–1914* (Cambridge University Press Cambridge 1994).

Hunter, R. and MacAlpine, I. *Psychiatry for the Poor. 1851 Colney Hatch Asylum-Friern Hospital 1973: a medical and social history* (Dawsons London 1974).

Ileto, R. 'Cholera and the origins of the American sanitary order in the Philippines', in D. Arnold, *Imperial Medicine and Indigenous Societies* (Oxford University Press New Delhi 1988).

Inden, R. *Imagining India* (Basil Blackwell Oxford 1990).

Inglis, B. *The Forbidden Game: a social history of drugs* (Hodder and Stoughton London 1975).

Jeffery, R. *The Politics of Health in India* (University of California London 1988).

Jeffery, R. and Jeffery, P. 'A Woman Belongs to Her Husband', in Alice Clark (ed.), *Gender and Political Economy: explorations of South Asian systems* (Oxford University Press New Delhi 1994).

Jordanova, L. 'The Social Construction of Medical Knowledge', in *Social History of Medicine*, 8, 1995.

Kakar, S. *Shamans, Mystics and Doctors: a psychological inquiry into India and its healing traditions* (Oxford University Press New Delhi 1982).

Keane, W. 'From Fetishism to Sincerity: on agency, the speaking subject and their historicity in the context of religious conversion', in *Comparative Study of Society and History*, 39, 1997.

King, A. *Colonial Urban Development: culture, social power and environment* (Routledge London 1976).

Lee, Y. 'Lunatics and Lunatic Asylums in early Singapore 1819–1869', in *Medical History* 19, 1973.

Lyons, M. *The Colonial Disease: a social history of sleeping sickness in northern Zaire 1900–1940* (Cambridge University Press Cambridge 1992).

Lyons, M. 'The Power to Heal: African medical auxiliaries in colonial Belgian Congo and Uganda', in D. Engels and S. Marks (eds), *Contesting Colonial hegemony: state and society in Africa and India* (British Academic Press 1994).

MacKenzie, C. *Psychiatry for the Rich: a history of the Private Ticehurst Asylum, 1792–1917* (Routledge London 1992).

MacLeod, R. and Lewis, M. (eds), *Disease, Medicine and Empire: perspectives on Western medicine and the experience of European expansion* (Routledge London 1988).

MacMillan, M. 'Anglo-Indians and the Civilizing Mission 1880–1914', in G. Krishna (ed.), *Contributions to South Asian Studies 2* (Oxford University Press New Delhi 1982).

Majeed, J. *Ungoverned Imaginings: James Mill's 'History of British India' and Orientalism* (Clarendon Press Oxford 1992).

Major-Poetzl, P. *Michel Foucault's Archaeology of Western Culture: toward a new science of history* (Harvester Brighton 1983).

Malcolm, E. *Swift's Hospital: a story of St. Patrick's Hospital, Dublin 1746–1989* (Gill and Macmillan Dublin 1989)

Mathur, L. *Kala Pani: history of Andaman and Nicobar Islands with a study of India's Freedom Struggle* (Eastern Books Delhi 1985).

Matthews, J. *Good and Mad Women: the historical construction of femininity in twentieth-century Australia* (Allen and Unwin St. Leonards 1984).

Mattlock, J. *Scenes of Seduction: prostitution, hysteria and reading difference in nineteenth-century France* (Columbia University Press New York 1994).

Metcalf, T. *The Aftermath of Revolt: India 1857–1870* (Princeton University Press Princeton 1965).

Metcalf, T. *Ideologies of the Raj* (Cambridge University Press Cambridge 1994).

Monk, J. 'Cleansing their Souls: laundries in institutions for fallen women', in *Lilith*, 9, 1996.

Monk, L. 'Working like Mad: nineteenth century female lunatic asylum attendants and violence', in *Lilith*, 9, 1996.

Nandy, A. *The Intimate Enemy: loss and recovery of self under colonialism* (Oxford University Press New Delhi 1983).

Nigam, S. 'Disciplining and policing the "criminals" by birth, Part I: the making of a colonial stereotype – the criminal tribes of North India', in *Indian Economic and Social History Review*, 27, 1990.

O'Hanlon, R. 'Recovering the Subject: Subaltern Studies and histories of resistance in colonial South Asia', in *Modern Asian Studies*, 22, 1, 1988.

Oldenburg, V. *The Making of Colonial Lucknow 1856–1877* (Oxford University Press New Delhi 1989).

Ortner, S. 'Resistance and the Problem of Ethnographic Refusal', in *Comparative Study of Society and History*, 37, 1995.

Panigrahi, L. *British Social Policy and Female Infanticide in India* (Munshiram Manoharlal New Delhi 1972).

Parker, R. *et al.*, 'County of Lancaster Asylum, Rainhill: 100 years ago and now', in *History of Psychiatry*, 4, 1993.

Parssinen, T. and Kerner, K. 'Development of the Disease Model of Drug Addiction in Britain 1870–1926', in *Medical History*, 24, 1980.

Pathak, Z. and Rajan, R. 'Shahbano', in *Signs*, 14, 1989.

Paul, J. 'Medicine and Imperialism', in J. Ehrenreich (ed.), *The Cultural Crisis of Modern Medicine* (Monthly Review Press New York 1978).

Paular, R. 'Mental Illness as a Social Problem in the Phillipines during the Spanish Colonial Period', in *Phillipine Journal of Psychology*, 25, 1992.

Persaud, R. 'A comparison of symptoms recorded from the same patients by an asylum doctor and a "Constant Observer" in 1823: the implications for theories about psychological illness in history', in *History of Psychiatry*, 3, 1992.

Persaud, R. 'The Reporting of Psychiatric Symptoms in History: the memorandum book of Samuel Coates 1785–1925', in *History of Psychiatry*, 4, 1993.

Peters, D. 'The British Medical Response to Opiate addiction in the nineteenth century', in *Journal of the History of Medicine and Allied Sciences*, xxxvi, 1981.

Porter, R. *A Social History of Madness: stories of the insane* (Weidenfeld and Nicolson London 1987).

Quétel, C. (translated by J. Braddock and B. Pike), *History of Syphilis* (Polity Press 1990).

Radhakrishna, M. 'The Criminal Tribes Act in Madras Presidency: implications for itinerant trading communities', in *Indian Economic and Social History Review*, 26, 1989.

Raghavan, V. *Law of Crimes: a single volume commentary on Indian Penal Code 1860 (Act no. 45 of 1860)* (Orient Law House New Delhi 1993).

Ray, L. 'Models of Madness in Victorian asylum practice', in *Archives Européennes de Sociologie*, 22, 1981.

Renvoize, E. and Beveridge, A. 'Mental Illness and the late Victorians: a study of patients admitted to three asylums in York 1880–1884', in *Psychological Medicine*, 19, 1989.

Ripa, Y. (translated by Catherine du Peloux Menagé), *Women and Madness: the incarceration of women in nineteenth-century France* (Polity Press Cambridge 1990).

Risse, G. and Warner, J. 'Reconstructing Clinical Activities: patient records and medical history', in *Social History of Medicine*, 5, 1992.

Rollin, H. 'Whatever happened to Henry Maudsley?', in G. Berrios and H. Freeman (eds), *150 Years of British Psychiatry 1841–1991* (Gaskell London 1991).

Rose, N. *The Psychological Complex: psychology, politics and society in England 1869–1939* (Routledge London 1985).

Rose, N. 'Calculable minds and manageable individuals', in *History of Human Sciences*, 1, 1988.

Rothman, D. *The Discovery of the Asylum: social order and disorder in the New Republic* (Little Brown Boston 1971).

Russell, R. 'The lunacy profession and its staff in the second half of the nineteenth century, with special reference to the West Riding Lunatic Asylum', in W. Bynum, R. Porter and M. Shepherd (eds), *The Anatomy of Madness: essays in the history of psychiatry*, vol. III (Routledge London 1988).

Salgado, G. *The Elizabethan Underworld* (J. Dent London 1977).

Saunders, J. 'Magistrates and Madmen: segregating the criminally insane in late nineteenth-century Warwickshire' in V. Bailey (ed.), *Policing and Punishment in Nineteenth-Century Britain* (Croom Helm London 1981).

Scott, J. *Weapons of the Weak: everyday forms of peasant resistance* (Yale University Press New Haven 1985).

Scull, A. *Museums of Madness: the social organisation of insanity in nineteenth-century England* (Penguin 1982).

Scull, A. 'Humanitarianism or Control? Some observations on the historiography of Anglo-American psychiatry', in S. Cohen and A. Scull (eds), *Social Control and the State: historical and comparative essays* (Blackwell Oxford 1985).

Scull, A. *Social Order/Mental Disorder: Anglo-American psychiatry in historical perspective* (Routledge London 1989).

Scull, A. *The Asylum as Utopia: W.A.F. Browne and the mid-nineteenth century consolidation of psychiatry* (Routledge London 1991).

Scull, A. *The Most Solitary of Afflictions: madness and society in Britain, 1700–1900* (Yale University Press London 1993).

Sharma, S. *Mental Hospitals in India* (Directorate General of Health Services New Delhi 1990).

Sheridan, R. *Doctors and Slaves: a medical and demographic history of slavery in the British West Indies 1680–1834* (Cambridge University Press Cambridge 1985).

Short, S. *Victorian Lunacy: Richard M. Bucke and the practice of late nineteenth-century psychiatry* (Cambridge University Press Cambridge 1986).

Showalter, E. *The Female Malady: women, madness and English culture, 1830–1980* (Virago London 1987).

Skaria, A. 'Writing, Orality and Power in the Dangs, Western India, 1800s–1920' in *Subaltern Studies IX* (Oxford University Press New Delhi 1997).

Slack, P. *Poverty and Policy in Tudor and Stuart England* (Longman London 1988).

Smith, R. *Trial by Medicine: insanity and responsibility in Victorian trials* (Edinburgh University Press Edinburgh 1981).

Stewart, L. 'The Edge of Utility: slaves and smallpox in the early eighteenth-century', in *Medical History*, 29, 1985.

Stokes, E. *The English Utilitarians and India* (Oxford University Press New Delhi 1959).

Swartz, S. 'The Black Insane in the Cape, 1891–1920', in *Journal of Southern African Studies*, 21, 1995.

Swartz, S. 'Changing Diagnoses in Valkenberg Asylum, Cape Colony 1891–1920', in *History of Psychiatry*, 6, 1995.

Swartz, S. 'Colonizing the insane: causes of insanity in the Cape, 1891–1920', in *History of the Human Sciences*, 8, 1995.

Thomas, N. *Colonialism's Culture: anthropology, travel and government* (Polity Press Oxford 1994).

R. Tolen, 'Colonizing and Transforming the Criminal Tribesman: the Salvation Army in British India', in J. Urla and J. Terry (eds), *Deviant Bodies: critical perspectives on difference in science and popular culture* (Indiana University Press Bloomington 1995).

Tomes, N. *A Generous Confidence. Thomas Story Kirkbride and the art of asylum keeping 1840–1883* (Cambridge University Press Cambridge 1984).

Turner, T. 'Schizophrenia as a Permanent Problem', *History of Psychiatry*, 3, 1992.

Urla, J. and Terry, J., *Deviant Bodies: critical perspectives on difference in science and popular culture* (Indiana University Press Bloomington 1995)

Vaughan, M. *Curing their Ills: colonial power and African illness* (Polity Press Oxford 1991).

Walker, N. *Crime and Insanity in England: the historical perspective* (Volume I) (Edinburgh University Press Edinburgh 1972).

Walker, N. and McCabe, S. *Crime and Insanity in England: new solutions and new problems*, Volume II (Edinburgh University Press Edinburgh 1973).

Walton, J. (ed.), *Brain's Diseases of the Nervous System 10th Edition* (Oxford University Press Oxford 1993).

Watson, S. 'Malingerers, the "weak-minded" criminal and the "moral imbecile" : how the English prison medical officer became an expert in mental deficiency, 1880–1930', in M. Clark and C. Crawford (eds), *Legal Medicine in History* (Cambridge University Press Cambridge 1994).

Waxler, N. 'Is Mental Illness Cured in Traditional Societies? A Theoretical Analysis', in *Culture, Medicine and Psychiatry*, 1, 1977.

White, H. *Tropics of Discourse: essays in cultural criticism* (Johns Hopkins University Press Baltimore 1978).

Wright, D. 'Getting Out of the Asylum: understanding the confinement of the insane in the nineteenth-century', in *Social History of Medicine*, 10, 1997.

Wright, D. 'The Certification of Insanity in Nineteenth-Century England and Wales', in *History of Psychiatry*, 9, 1998.

Yang, A. *Crime and Criminality in British India* (University of Arizona Press Tucson 1985).

Zastoupil, L. *John Stuart Mill and India* (Stanford University Press Stanford 1994).

Index